From The Inside Out

Anna Anderson

From The Inside Out
© Anna Anderson Ltd
2021

Anna Anderson Ltd.
www.annaandersoninc.com

Copy editing by Esther Goh and Casandra Farren
Book production by Bogdan Matei
Front cover design by Margo Bobrowicz
Author photography Becky Rui

ISBN: Paperback 978-1-5262-0901-6

To Isaac – the best teacher I have ever had –
and Mike, the person who saw me before I saw myself.
Thank you always my loves.

"Love is the answer. You can search the entire universe for someone who is more deserving of your love and affection than you are yourself, and that person is not to be found anywhere. You yourself, as much as anyone in the entire universe, deserve your love and affection."

- Buddha

Praise for
From The Inside Out

This book is beautiful, it moved my soul, it reached the core of me. - **Yvonne Sutton**

Only starting chapter 3 but oh how amazing are we?. Already given me that first wake up call I desperately needed and written out what I need to give my body and what I'm thankful for it for. Excited for what's to come next. - **Lorraine Cameron**

Reading your book was like FINALLY finding the light switch and turning the light on in my head (I'm 53 years old!). I made an immediate change to care for and love myself every day. I stopped immediately (and I mean it) thinking negative thoughts about myself and tearing myself to pieces. It really works! I feel better, I look better and I walk around with my back straight and feeling proud. When I realised how I had been treating myself I was ashamed that I had done that for so many years, but I'm making up for that from now on and for the rest of my life. Thank you Anna. - **Sigurlaug Val Sigvaldadóttir**

Wow, so much amazing info and insight. My heart and mind are feeling calmer and hopeful for the first time in ages, I will continue to read it often and watch out for your words of wisdom in your group - thank you Anna.
- Veronica Gallen

I've just finished reading your book. I know beyond doubt that I will be returning to it regularly. You have helped me to recognise that despite working hard to overcome health issues and depression, that I still have some serious self-worth hang ups that are preventing me from moving forward with my ambitions to turn my creative hobby into a business. At no time has it ever occurred to me to learn to love every bit of me and to nurture my physical body. And then, with the will of God, perhaps I will feel more deserving and learn to fly in my business dreams too. Thank you so much for sharing your story and advice. Best wishes
- Mary-Ann Toop

I've just finished reading your book, it was so enlightening! Thank you. Biggest revelation is that self love does not come from going to the hairdresser or nail bar, which everyone tells me I should be doing to get some me time but I hate doing, instead from taking the time to do things like prepare the fresh food, take a walk etc all of which I like doing! - **Sarah Wood**

I have just finished reading your book. Wow it's absolutely spot on. I love your story and how you came to write the book. This is just what I needed over the past 3 years I have been through a lot of changes which my inner voice has absolutely loved!!! - **Jennie Rowe**

From a place of darkness, grief, illness, fear and anxiety, this book has set me on a path of light, freedom, health, confidence, laughter and most of all love. I can't praise the work of Anna enough. From impressive, knowledgeable health and nutritional advice to deep psychological understanding and support, Anna really does help to alter your mindset and set you on a path of gentle nurturing, self care and love. Thank you so much Anna, you really have given me my life back! xx - **Clare Willoughby**

I had lived for decades stuck in a downward spiral of bingeing, purging and starvation diets. Living a life stuck in shame that I was such a failure. I didn't know how to feel normal and really felt that I had completely lost the battle. I felt that I didn't know me - I knew who I had to pretend to be to function in my life - but I was hiding so much that I was just exhausted from the effort and terrified of being so out of control. Then I found Anna's book online. I couldn't believe that someone seemed to know what I was feeling - after all these years of self hatred, guilt and shame this came as a complete revelation - it wasn't just me! I could finally see that there might be a way out. I devoured the book and went on to work with Anna on her Nuture and Nourish programme. I've learned so much about myself and found the confidence to let others in. I'm sharing previously buried thoughts, feelings and experiences and finally feel that I am living life as the authentic me. I don't have those dark corners where shame and guilt can continue to punish me. I am discovering more everyday about what I need. I have tools to help me manage overwhelm, stress and anxiety. I know how to find out what I'm actually feeling and how to listen to myself. I have had wobbles, but even then I know that that's OK , life is a journey and I don't have to be perfect. I am living a much more calm and peaceful life. From the bottom of my heart Anna, I would like to thank you for showing me that there is another way to happiness within - that doesn't involve diets, deprivation, wagons, yo-yo's or using self hatred as a weapon to beat myself into submission to be 'good'. It has been incredibly freeing to learn that it is not about food, diets or deprivation. I still have a lot of work to do and cannot wait to continue on my journey. I started out thinking what I wanted to say about Anna's book - just read it, it will change your life. It's definitely changed mine. **- Julie Callaway**

Clicking on the link for your page was the most life-changing thing I have ever done. I read your ebook that night and immediately knew I needed to change my self-criticism and start to finally love all of myself and know I was worthy. Working with you on the 8wk course was the icing on the cake. It's changed my life in so many ways and given me tools to use forever. Thank you Anna! xx **- Jane Edwards**

I was obviously meant to meet Anna when I came across her book in October 2020 and chaos was everywhere in my life. I had been very poorly and on lots of medication.

Anna not only taught me how to feed my body with what it needed to be well but how to stop playing myself the same old self-destruct tune. I had spent 30 years being so unkind to myself. I transformed my eating and I retrained and changed my career after finally learning to believe in myself. I no longer need migraine medication, and my blood pressure has returned to normal. I have so much to thank Anna for, the words just don't seem enough. I have also made the most amazing lifelong friends. Forever grateful! xxx - **Cathy Waiton**

Reading 'From The Inside Out' was like a penny dropping - the missing link to my happiness. It just makes the most perfect sense, small changes that make the most profound and life-changing differences. Thank you Anna from the bottom of my heart. - **Jenny Parry**

A sense of calm washed over me as I finished Anna's book and I said to myself 'finally'. Thank you Anna! - **Angie Martin**

Years of doing dieting resulted in temporary fixes, increased self-damage, and only tapped away at the outside surface, the symptom, not the cause. Connecting with Anna Anderson in January 2021 has changed my world and now I am growing by slowing. Integrity and openness have powered my growth. With each day, I feel more energy, alive and enormously grateful for Anna's wise, gentle, and loving guidance. Anna's extended group coaching programme has supported me in being, increasing my awareness, uncovering, and understanding who I am, my past wounds, thoughts and beliefs and have led me on a journey towards self-understanding, love, and acceptance. I'm on my way back to myself and with each day I experience increased self-connection, freedom and I'm feeling alive again. I'm ready for and so want this healing journey to continue. Heartfelt thanks Anna, I am forever grateful. Love! - **Emma H**

Anna's teaching is life changing. After years of undervaluing myself, putting myself below everybody else's needs, talking negatively about myself to myself, and feeling like I'd completely lost my identity, Anna was a ray of light. Passionate about what she does, she makes you feel like you again; makes you think differently about yourself; brings you light, love, happiness, self acceptance, confidence, and so much more. Working with her has been the best thing I have ever done. I love being me! It's absolutely amazing! Thank you Anna. You are a bright shining star. - **Sally Alexander**

Contents

My Naked Truth

As I sit here at my desk, wondering how to begin writing this, my eyes well with tears. Reconnecting with the woman I was at the beginning of this journey and how she was feeling fills me with deep sadness for her and how lost she was. I wonder what she would think of the woman I have become as a result of the huge shifts in my life through learning to love myself from the inside out. Back then, I would have loved for someone to scoop me up and show me what to do. My intention is for this book to serve in that role for you: a warm and safe place for you to learn how to not only nourish yourself but realise you are truly worthy of your own love.

If you are struggling with starting a diet every Monday or even every day; if you are tired of deciding you will 'be good' in the morning and finding it has all gone out the window by the afternoon; if you are tired of looking in the mirror and hating what you see; if you are tired of worrying about what you look like, what you said, what you ate; and if there is a knowing within you that you are more than this and there must be a different, more peaceful way, then this is for you. I see you, I understand, and believe me, you are not alone. You are in the right place. There is another way to live, which I will share with you here in these pages - along with some insights into why this pattern seems so obviously simple to overcome yet feels impossibly hard.

I will start by sharing my story, my naked truth. My hope is it stirs something deep within you; a hope, an inspiration, or the rumblings of a new belief that you can indeed change your life and have everything you have been searching for. You are not stuck. What you desire is entirely achievable. It might just be that what you have been searching for all this time lies somewhere else entirely. Perhaps it is simply time to take a new path.

I am not sure exactly when I hit rock bottom. I think there was a series of many, or perhaps I was just scraping along the bottom for a very long time. I had been receiving a continuous calling to listen and make change but at the time I wasn't conscious enough to know what was happening. Sometimes we are so good at ignoring those callings that it takes a very powerful and rocky awakening before we actually do anything about them! I was very good at consistently ignoring my own instincts and in response I had the rug well and truly pulled out from underneath my feet.

One of the rock bottoms that sticks out in my mind is one sunny Saturday in July 2014 when I consumed the best part of a bottle of gin by 10.30am, so let's start there.

On that particular day I had waved my four-year-old son off to his dad's for the weekend and as I closed the door, the loneliness and pain I'd come to know so well washed over me. It had all become too much for me to bear and the only answer I could find was to numb the pain with alcohol, food, shopping, and being busy. I needed a constant stream of distractions in my life because sitting with the pain was unbearable – if I stayed busy, I didn't need to address any of it.

I had ticked all of the external boxes I had been taught would make me happy. I had done well at school, managed to scrape through college, went to university, went travelling, got a good job, and by the time of the gin incident I was 32 years old and working in London for a software company.

While all looked good on the surface, there was also a deep emptiness within me. One which, if I am honest, I probably didn't even know was there at the time. I just knew I wasn't happy. But I also thought this was life – this was all there was. I drank heavily – more heavily than I would like to admit, but working in the city as a single woman in her 20s I could get away with it because it was a normalised behaviour. Dinner regularly consisted of a bottle of Sauvignon. I had been drinking since I was 14 years old, hanging around with people older than me, doing things you definitely wouldn't want your teenage daughter to be doing. Looking back, I can see there were times I was in real danger. I am lucky I got away with as much as

I did and lived to tell the tale. And I now realise these feelings and numbing patterns started from a very young age.

I was almost always the most drunk at a party. Regularly legless. Deeply concerned with my body image and what I looked like. Consumed by self-judgement and criticism and deeply ashamed of who I was. I constantly sought approval from others, because my self-perception was based heavily on what everyone else thought. I was a people pleaser and desperately wanted to be liked and accepted.

I believed all would be well when I finally looked a certain way or weighed in at a specific number. I believed weight loss came through restriction and starving myself, yet food was one of the only pleasures I had. I lived in a constant polarity of starving, numbing and feeling guilt and shame.

I tried every diet under the sun. I binged, I purged, I took diet pills. I looked in the mirror and hated what I saw. I felt guilty when I ate. I pinched my body and wished I could cut off the bits I hated. I looked at other women with envy and compared my size against other people in photos. I had no concept of what I looked like – I absolutely believed I was fat and ugly, even though I can now see that was not the case. (So many women I speak to feel the same way. They realise in hindsight how beautiful they really were but just didn't feel able to connect with that at the time.)

The wheels were sure to come off. It was simply a matter of time. The gentle rumblings the Universe had consistently been sending my way, urging me to listen to myself, had not been enough. I was definitely going to need more of a nudge, and that happened for me in the shape of my beautiful son, Isaac. My world shifted in the most unexpected way when I became single and pregnant at 28…I was about to face the very real wake-up call I needed.

I was immediately in love with the baby growing inside of me. But I had absolutely no concept of the responsibility of parenthood or the challenges and pressures of being a single Mum. I was about to find out!

My pregnancy went by with ease. I was so excited to meet my son, and on 17th October 2010, at 7.32pm, my beautiful baby boy came into the world. Isaac has been a profound teacher for me, teaching me patience and the truth of unconditional love.

For a while we got by OK. I took maternity leave and went back to my job. It was really tough to balance it all.

One day, Isaac needed nappies and my card was declined at the shop. I was so ashamed. I couldn't even afford to provide for my son. That was one of my lowest points.

Isaac started going to visit his Dad and stay overnight long before either of us were ready, which I struggled with enormously. I hated the weekends he went away – I wasn't sure who I was supposed to be. I didn't get invited to things with other parents and I didn't want to go back to my partying days with friends who didn't have children because I didn't feel they 'got it'. I no longer knew who I was or where my place in the world was. In my struggle to figure out my new identity, I felt so lost, alone, and confused. The loneliness, judgement, shame, and sadness were overwhelming. I was also terrified of dying and expected to get sick and leave Isaac alone and helpless at any point.

Four years in, everything was spiralling out of control. I was juggling a corporate job I was no longer enjoying, exhausted by trying to manage it all. I could no longer be everything to everyone. Commuting three hours a day and a son who'd still never slept a full night had taken its toll. I was drinking heavily and using food to comfort myself. I remember being frightened of going to bed without having at least one or two glasses of wine first because I no longer knew how to go to sleep sober. I thought I knew what it meant to eat healthily but really I had no idea, with so much confusing information out there and a desire to be thin over healthy. I would wake up every day, weigh myself and hope I looked thin when I looked in the mirror. But I was overweight, puffy around the face, and seeing photos of myself made me so very sad.

Unhealthy and unfit, running up the stairs would leave me breathless. I had absolutely no energy from day to day. I felt so low, totally disconnected from my body, and apart from time with my son, I just didn't like life very much. When I looked around at everyone else, they seemed to have it all together, like life was effortlessly great for them. For me, just getting through the day was a struggle.

But the day after I cracked open that bottle of gin, nursing the usual hangover, something deep within me stirred and a voice said, "You have so much more to share with the world than this. You can do and be so much more to Isaac, so much more to yourself." These words have stayed with me ever since – perhaps I could be my own knight in shining armour after all? Scrap that. I didn't need a man to come and save me – I could be my own Goddess Warrior. I could make the change I was so desperately seeking. I realised I needed to do something different, although I had absolutely no idea what different looked like. I still felt completely stuck, but something within me had shifted and I knew I couldn't carry on as I was.

I decided the first place to start was giving up my job. By this time I had moved to Haslemere in Surrey and I was still working in London. The commute was killing me and Isaac was about to go to school. If I had kept that job, I would have had to pay someone to be with him before and after school, and I would only see him at the weekends. I was not prepared to miss out on this time with the most precious thing in my life. So, I decided to hand in my notice.

This was a big decision. I was a single Mum and at that time, didn't believe I had any other skills. I had based a lot of my identity and worth in the fact that at least I had a 'good job' so giving that up terrified me.

Sitting in bed on the Sunday after the gin incident, once again nursing a hangover and dreading Monday, I googled 'jobs for Mums'. The first thing that came up in my search was a link about buying a yoga teaching franchise. It said – 'great opportunity for Mums to run a business around their family'. There was a phone number to discuss the opportunity further.

Something attracted me to the idea. Looking back, I see that everything happens for a reason. I was being guided to a very different path but I was going to have to be very brave if I wanted to make a different life for myself and my son.

Before we go any further, let's be clear. I was not a yoga teacher nor indeed had I done much yoga. I was not in any form of physical shape. I had never before done a downward dog. I had never run my own business. I believed I was rubbish with money – often filling the emptiness inside with a spending splurge. Any money I did have, I frittered away, hence the nappy incident. I also had a deeply ingrained belief that I was not sporty. P.E. for me had been a horrendous experience – I remember being picked on for my pale legs, standing out on the school field in the freezing cold and hating every moment of it.

Starting my own business, teaching yoga – when I knew nothing about either of those things – was neither a sensible nor wise move, especially as the sole provider. Yet my heart was whispering, 'You can do this, this is for you'. It was downright crazy, but I reached a point where I was so desperate for something to change I was prepared to do whatever it took.

While I am not suggesting you leave a job you hate right now, what I will say is you need to show up for yourself and make brave moves that scare you. Transformation happens outside of your comfort zone. For me, that is what being alive is: trusting the Universe has something truly great in store for each of us (because it does if you allow it!). The more we surrender to that path and trust it, taking steps into the unknown without needing evidence of how it is going to turn out, the more we are supported. Life is way too short to do something you hate doing to create a seemingly successful life whilst you are silently dying on the inside.

I called the number. Within an hour I had bought a yoga franchise on my credit card. There was no turning back. I went to work the following day and handed in my notice. I left my 'safe' city job and went on a quest to not only learn how to be a yoga teacher, but also how to build a business and earn enough to provide for my little family. Little did I know at the time what yoga was about to do for me!

I credit two things for changing my world, Isaac and yoga. My son taught me I needed to show up for myself, to love myself in order to be able to be the mother he deserved. If I wanted him to be able to stand in his strength and wisdom and love himself unconditionally, I would need to be able to model that for him. Whatever I wanted to give him, I had to give to myself first. It required me to step up and do the inner work. To look within and become a better version of myself. Those low moments – the gin, the not being able to buy nappies – were the very wake-up calls I needed to pull me out of my own victimhood and realise I was the only one who was ever going to come and save me. Yoga gave me the tools to find all of the wisdom inside of myself. It gave me the internal awareness and space I needed to learn how to build a loving relationship with myself. But if you had told me that at the time I probably would have scoffed and told you to buy me another glass of wine!

For me, yoga was the doorway to transformation. In the space I made for myself on that mat I tuned into the truth of who I was. I had been searching outside of myself for such a long time to fill the emptiness, to be enough, to be loveable. I had numbed the pain with alcohol, food, shopping, and drugs. Through the practice of yoga I learned I had been looking in the wrong places to feel full. The answers were within me. I had been ignoring myself, my soul, my knowing, my inner voice. The whole time she was there – loving me, whispering to me. The love and worthiness I had been seeking was available – I just needed to give it to myself. On my mat I learned to honour myself. I learned to love my body – that my body is my home. I learned to slow down and listen to my soul. What I had been seeking was inside of me. All I needed to do was slow down and tune in.

One of the great yoga teachers BKS Iyengar said, "Yoga does not change the way we see things, it transforms the person who sees." For me, this could not be more true.

I gained so much wisdom through my yoga practice that I applied to my life. It is about the journey, not the destination. My heart was full of wisdom I had never listened to before. The more I practised, the more my self-awareness developed. I could see how I had been treating myself; that I had been looking outside of myself for what was actually within me. The more I moved and connected to my body, the more I wanted to take care of it.

At the time, I lived in a tiny 18th-century house. You could reach out and touch both sides of the galley kitchen, which had just enough room to put a yoga mat on the floor. It was literally the only space I had, so that's where I practised yoga every day. All of a sudden, I had a purpose! Something to work on, I could see myself getting better at. I would wake up early every day so that I could practice before the day got busy. I started to feel better. I had more energy. My body was getting stronger, I felt more confident. And I found myself naturally wanting to make different lifestyle choices. I didn't want to drink any more because I wanted to get up early to practice. I became fascinated by food and what was healthy for my body. I started reading and studying, and I felt excited for the first time in a long time.

The more I made little changes, the better I felt. I was no longer doing things for external validation, but for myself and my son. I noticed the presence of foreign feelings like peace, joy, and contentment. One day I looked in the mirror and realised I looked completely different. The swelling and puffiness had gone and I had lost weight without trying – simply by taking care of myself. It was what my body had wanted all along and it came from nourishing myself and taking small, aligned action every day.

My little yoga business slowly grew. I really put the work in: I went to fetes and events and connected with as many people as I could. I did things completely out of my comfort zone and my inner critic was often screaming *NOOOOO, THIS IS WAY TOO SCARY!* But I did it anyway and it was always OK.

My first yoga class had just two people in it, and one of those spaces I had given as a gift! But I didn't give up, and I didn't let fear take over. You might be wondering how I managed to make it work financially as a single parent; I had a small amount of savings to tide us over for a couple of months, Isaac's father paid child maintenance to support him, and I lived very carefully. Even though I felt worried a lot of the time, I learned to rein in my fear when she got loud. I created a mantra to use when anxiety hit. "Today you have everything you need, today you have enough." I believed if I stayed positive and focussed on where I wanted to go, it would all be alright.

What I have learned about money is that the right mindset is essential. If you focus on what you lack and spend time caught up in fear and worry, it will create more of the same. I now see money as a beautiful enabling energy that allows me to create and serve in the world. I even celebrate and practice appreciation when I pay my tax bill – believe me, that one took a while! Your relationship with money is deeply connected to your relationship with food, your body, and ultimately your self-worth. These aspects are all intrinsically linked and as you come home to yourself you will notice healing in many areas – not just food. By committing to elevating your financial situation you are committing to expansion. The world is not served by you staying stuck with limited financial resources; with more money, you can help more people. Money in the hands of women, the world's nurturers, is an important part of our global healing. And when you commit to your own expansion in all senses of the word, everyone in your life benefits from your improved well-being on all fronts.

Over time, my classes grew and grew. It was a really special time. Not only had I set up my own business, but I was also managing to support my son, and spend the time with him that he needed, all while helping people too – it was a perfect combination. I loved what I was doing so much. Where there was once fear and sadness, my heart started to fill with joy and appreciation.

I was taking down the walls and softening into my truth.

And then my life really started to change.

For most of my life, my relationships with men had not been very successful. I now realise this stemmed from a deep lack of self-worth: a deep fear of not being good enough and of being left. This resulted in choosing men who were either not good enough (who were either never going to treat me well or stick around) or running away from the nice guys (I believed if I let them in and they saw my truth, they would leave me). This pattern was driven by a subconscious attempt at self-preservation. *Stay alone and you won't get hurt.* I kept making choices that hurt me and gave me even more evidence I wasn't good enough.

But this new me had started to love who she was. Prior to this I wanted to be in a relationship to feel seen, to feel loved, and feel enough. I didn't need that anymore. I was learning I could give this to myself. At one point I very clearly remember thinking *I don't need to meet anyone anymore. If I do, great, but I am not prepared to compromise – they have to be exceptional!* One month later I met my husband, Mike; the most conscious, emotionally aware and open man I have ever met. He had done his work. It felt like it was meant to be and very quickly we fell in love.

During this time, I had been growing my yoga business and in teaching women yoga, I noticed some patterns in the way we treat ourselves and the beliefs we hold. I realised I wasn't the only one who had been feeling the way I was. It was consistent in many women who came to my classes. I also realised that one yoga class a week was not going to be enough to help these women make radical change and learn to love who they are in the way I wanted to show them.

I decided to build an online program to teach other women the things I had learned that had made such a difference in my life. The only problem was, I had no idea how! While on holiday with my brother in Thailand in April 2017, I shared my vision and ambition with him. At this point I had no awareness of how the Universe is always listening and always supporting us if we ask! The next month, I met Mike and it just so happened he knew of a course that would teach me how to create my vision and bring it to life.

In order to do this course, I needed £10,000, which I didn't have. I borrowed it from my mum and stepdad, who had supported me so much by this point, I felt really embarrassed to ask, especially for something that wasn't exactly a sure bet. But I signed up and took the plunge. All of a sudden I was swept into a sea of unknowns. I was WAY out of my comfort zone in this new world of coaches and experts, and that eight-week course was the most terrifying thing I had done to date. But I showed up and kept putting the work in. I learned technical systems and concepts I had never heard of, and over a few months built a program that was ready to share. This was the birth of The Nurture and Nourish System™ that has now reached women all around the world.

To start with, I tested it on a few people. Would they enjoy it? Would it work? And it did – it served and made a beautiful difference to the women who had come through it. That gave me hope and fuelled my belief that what I had to share could help even more people.

That program grew legs and it dawned on me that I needed to become a professional coach if I truly wanted to help others - something I had never even considered before! I realised I had been coaching myself and I was now starting to coach these ladies, so I needed to know how to do it properly. I trained as a Life Coach, Health Coach, NLP and EFT Practitioner, and am still continuously learning about why we do what we do, our unconscious conditioning and how to create freedom in our lives.

People often ask me how I got from where I was back then to where I am now and my answer is always that I showed up for myself first. Every day I have taken a step towards shining my light more brightly, feeling the discomfort and fear and doing it anyway, healing myself, learning and growing. I have gotten clear on my values and if something doesn't align, I don't do it. I have been disciplined, I have let go of relationships that haven't been working, I have committed fully to myself – to leaning into fear and learning how to fully love and accept all parts of myself. This work will never be done and that excites me! I have realised I am a continuous project and I intend to be a new person each day.

I have learned to let go of control and instead trust and surrender. I haven't given mixed messages to the Universe – whilst I have been terrified, I have always been all in, and there has been no plan B. There were so many times

I wanted to give up, when it felt too hard, when I cried and thought 'I am going to get a job' – but I didn't. I kept going, day after day. My focus has always been making a difference to the women who are feeling the way I used to feel. I believe if we make the focus of our lives bigger than ourselves, the universe will always support us in bringing that into being. I want to see as many women as possible in their power because I know it is truly available to us all.

If I can get here, then you can find your way to your dream too. Seriously. That is why I have written this book. I see you before you see yourself, and sometimes that is all we need: a gentle and loving nudge away from the destructive cycles of body shaming, dieting and restriction, and the realisation it was only ever your own love you were seeking.

In order to create the life of your dreams, you might have to let go of a few of the stories and expectations you are carrying around about how you think things 'should' be. I remember how much I hated Isaac going to visit his Dad. The one thing in my life which brought me joy went away every other weekend and I didn't know if he was OK over there, or any of the things a Mum needs to know about her children. I felt like I was failing him, I felt like a bad Mum, and I felt like there was a part of me missing. Then a time came when I realised it was not the situation which was making me unhappy, it was in fact how I chose to see it. I was creating my own suffering by clinging to the fact I wanted it to be different, and that I didn't want him to go.

If I wanted to be happy, I had to accept that. Suddenly, everything became much easier.

You have to let go of your idea of 'how' you want things to be, and move forward towards the wonders that are waiting for you.

Whilst it might be challenging to hear, you are responsible for your life experience. Yes – sometimes we get dealt tough lessons. People regularly face deep and painful challenges. But I have learned that if I look at everything I experience as a gift then life becomes a much more joyful and graceful experience. Of course, we absolutely need to take time to process our experiences and believe me, some of those experiences are very hard, I truly respect that. However, I have realised, in reality, I have needed the lessons I've received in order to be able to grow and fulfil my potential.

Life is like the ocean. It is powerful, beautiful, serene, destructive and everything in between – you can either choose to be a pebble smashed around by it waiting to see where you are taken, or you can choose to build a ship and sail the oceans with confidence and courage. You know storms will come and that is OK – you also know you will gain strength and wisdom from them. If your ship is strong, you will get through it. You can master the storm, rather than feeling like a victim to it.

Your mind is your ship. Right now, your subconscious is most likely weakening your ability to sail the storm, full of mis-truths and stories which simply are not true. The exciting news is that you can change that.

Through the practice of looking within, doing the hard work and the self-enquiry, and learning to accept myself, I have truly never been happier. My message to you is this. You CAN have everything you desire but you don't have to DO everything. Achievement doesn't come from busyness and serving and pushing, ignoring your needs and dishonouring the parts of you that are calling to be seen, loved, and expressed. It comes from LOVING yourself. It comes from treating yourself with the love, nourishment, and self-care your soul has been longing for your whole life. It comes from listening to your Inner Knowing and trusting your Intuition. It comes from allowing yourself joy - finding what lights you up and making time to experience joy on a regular basis.

Look at the word Intuition. In Tuition. Your inner learning, your Inner Knowing. You truly have all of the answers to your own questions. Your job is to do yourself the honour of slowing down and listening to that tuition.

Allow yourself to move away from the masculine energy of doership which society has taught us is the only way and move to the feminine energy of connection, community and love. From there you can manifest all of your desires and live a very different life of health and vitality.

It all starts from the inside out.

Learn to love yourself from within. It is only from this place of kindness that you can start to achieve results on the outside too. Health is what it's all about - not weight loss. Learning to love and appreciate who you are, discovering how to take care of the great body that you live in, will get you the results that you've been dreaming of – inside and out.

You are worthy of so much more. Remember, the only person you need to show up for is you. You don't need to prove yourself to anyone. There is an inner calling within each and every one of us. This book is about learning how to listen to that calling. I believe we eat to comfort ourselves because we have been taught not to listen to the truth of who we are. My wish for you is that this book helps you reconnect with the beautiful, wise woman who sits within you, your inner Goddess…because the more you tune into her and love her, the more her voice will turn from a whisper into a roar. You have an innate power and capability that you might not have connected to fully before. But the more you show up for yourself, the more you honour yourself, forgive yourself and let go of the shackles and stories you have been weighing yourself down with, the more you will be able to trust who you came here to be.

So many of us are suffering; stuck in trauma, limiting beliefs, and unhealthy patterns. These behaviours are so deeply entrenched in modern society. How much time and space are we really giving ourselves to love who we are? How often do we have a negative internal dialogue? When were we taught that depression and anxiety are created by trauma held in our nervous system and that we can release them and heal?

Women have been taught for centuries that they are loveable only when they are of service to others and meet a socially acceptable physical expectation. We put our needs at the bottom of the pile and get stuck in shame and comparison. We fill that void with anything that might make us feel better; shopping, food, alcohol, or even unhealthy relationships.

The true goal is not weight loss, but self-love and acceptance. Many women come to me wanting to lose weight, but ultimately that is merely a symptom of a deeper root cause. Dieting is one of the most deeply damaging things a woman can do. It perpetuates the feelings of unworthiness and creates a shameful, disconnected relationship with the body. Most women I work with cannot even look in the mirror and hate taking photos of themselves. They diet to overcome this, the cycle continues, and the void deepens.

No amount of weight loss will make you more worthy. When the intention behind health comes from a place of self-love and nourishment, then true health naturally follows. Ridding ourselves of limiting beliefs and realising our worth is where healing really begins. Through these actions we not only start our individual healing, but we begin to heal the whole of female society.

You can change the beliefs that you hold. You are completely free. It may not feel like it right now, but I promise that you have the liberty to rewrite that map and draw a new one.

Often, we don't really know ourselves. We don't know what's going on in our subconscious; we're not even aware of our internal dialogue. Once we wake up to all of this, we can achieve massive transformation. Awareness is curative. We've got to get to know who we are in order to make a change, and to ultimately find happiness.

Looking back, I didn't even realise I had been feeling all of these things. I just got on with life in a very unconscious way without any awareness of how I was really feeling. The same patterns kept popping up, yet I never realised that I was unknowingly creating these cycles. Nor did I realise that the person I was looking for to save me was myself.

It is my mission to help guide women and transform their lives through a journey of self-discovery and healing. I am grateful to have now watched thousands of women achieve incredible results through my Nurture and Nourish™ system. Through the practice of self-love and acceptance, I help women step out of the shadow of years of dieting to achieve health and long-term weight loss.

So there is my story. Laid out bare – my naked truth. I share it with you to inspire. If there was hope for me, I promise there is hope for you. The question is simply –

are you ready? Are you ready to live the life intended for you?

Are you ready to break free from diets? To learn to nourish your body with life-giving foods? To throw your scales in the bin? To untie the shackles around your ankles and let go of the baggage weighing you down? To liberate yourself so that you can soar in the true expression of you without fear of judgement, without shame, and without the negative Nancy voiceover in your head?

If the answer is yes, then it is time for you to step into who you truly came here to be.

Life is waiting for you.

Buckle up, sister. Let's go on a ride together.

I am excited to soar with you!

Love, Anna x

P.S. There are a few things to know before you read any further.

1. This is not a typical diet book. It is not another one of those books telling you how to lose weight or what to eat. It guides you through all the reasons dieting isn't the answer and instead shows you how to build a loving relationship with yourself, which

in turn will support you in building a loving and joyful relationship with food.

2. I have designed this book to include lots of reader participation. I have not written it in chapters, but in sections, so that you can pick it up and put it down easily. At the end of each section there are suggested exercises and affirmations to use. They don't need to be followed in any specific order. Dip in and out; use them as much and often as you like. I suggest you start with the sections you feel most aligned with and create a toolbox of techniques to help you move through life. I have found the exercises I share profoundly life-changing. Give them a go and see how you feel. This is all about making the journey your own, so adapt and explore these ideas to find a way that feels right. Most importantly, enjoy it – bring a lightness to this work and see what comes up for you. The most important thing in healing is that you feel good so take this at your own pace.

3. It's a great idea to have a journal to hand as you read this book and keep it with you to note ideas and thoughts. I give you permission to treat yourself to a lovely journal that makes you happy! Make notes, observe your mind, notice what comes up...practice lots of self-enquiry. You are now your very own best detective!

Your Naked Truth

I have shared my journey with you from a place of vulnerability because I truly believe in the power of storytelling. We heal through sharing with each other and talking about our tough experiences, our hurts, our shame, our truths. We can connect and support each other. We learn that we are enough, that none of us are broken, that we can help each other and that there is nothing wrong with us. Shame is fostered by secrets. The more we share the more we realise we are not alone in our struggles.

Healing comes from within. You have everything you need to create freedom, joy and health in your life. So let's hand the reins over to you and your naked truth. I will walk by your side, cheering you on and guiding you back home to the truth of who you are.

You Are Enough

Your relationship with food and weight is not really about your relationship with food and weight. It is about your deep, raw, vulnerable, and very real need to be seen, loved, and understood.

It is a symptom of a deeper hunger.

The hunger to be loved and accepted and to know you are enough.

You are enough.

You always have been.

You are so deeply precious.

Your healing lies in your own realisation of how wonderful you are, just as you are now.

Your healing lies in love.

It lies within you.

It is found in your own love and acceptance.

As Carl Rogers wrote in his book On Becoming a Person: "The curious paradox is that when I accept myself just as I am, then I can change."

Unlike other books, this one will begin with the most important parts. I want to make reading this book as easy and enjoyable as possible. If you are anything like me, you have a pile of books you keep meaning to read by the side of your bed and I don't want this to be another one of them!

So, listen up – you were born for a reason. Your unique set of skills and talents are required in the world and you are already enough. This knowledge is the foundation upon which you can build the rest of your life.

It might not feel this way right now, but let me assure you it is the absolute truth. It is true for every single human on this planet and therefore I know it to be true for you too.

But what does this even mean? I am enough of what?! We see all of these memes flying around on social media with feel-good sentiments, but how can you feel enough when there is a deep sense of not enoughness (sometimes I make up words!) within you?

I never understood how being told 'I am enough' could possibly make me feel better because quite frankly, I didn't feel enough in any aspect of my life. I always interpreted it as - I should just be happy with my lot and not expect great things. I clearly wasn't enough because everyone else was out there living their best life!

What 'you are enough' actually means is you came into this world whole. You came in full of potential, full of wisdom, full of love. You are the only version of you. No one will ever walk this world in your likeness. Ever. That makes you remarkable, special and someone to absolutely be celebrated.

It means you do not need to prove your worth through anything you do. Simply being you, in all your light and glory, is enough. And from there you grow – sharing your light with the world.

The world isn't set up to teach us that we are worthy. In fact, the message tends to be the opposite – you are only worthy when you have proved it by meeting external expectations.

Enter the role of alcohol, food, sex, spending, gambling, drugs, born from a need to escape the very real pain of not being good enough.

But that is just not true.

You're beautiful enough. You're special enough. You're sexy, playful, and fun enough. You've worked enough. You've cried enough. You've been grateful, generous, and kind enough. You are enough.

In fact - you are more than enough. You are fabulous. Allow yourself to shine.

The more you allow yourself to move into this truth, the more you can put down the belief you will only be good enough when you achieve success in whatever way you measure it. The more you detach your worth from factors external to yourself, the more you realise you are perfectly imperfect and in actual fact, you can create the life of your dreams. You don't need to be anyone else, compare yourself to anyone else, or to prove your loveability. When you realise this you give yourself permission to go out there and set the world on fire.

What if you were born to thrive and it was your job to let go of the stories in your head that are preventing you from achieving the very things you desire? Let that marinate for a while...

You Are Unique and Remarkable

No-one has your laugh, your eyes, your handwriting, the complex tapestry of life experiences that have made you who you are – you are unique, individual, and remarkable. The only thing that limits you or keeps you stuck is your own disconnection from that truth. No one will ever walk this earth in your likeness ever again. That makes you so very special.

How can you compare yourself to others when you are the only version of you? There may well be lots of other humans on this planet but there isn't anyone in your likeness. There is little point trying to be someone else because that is impossible. But you can be the very best version of you! You are a very special individual indeed. You might have had a tough childhood, you might have had tough experiences...I hear you, but shaping your life around the past is not serving you or anyone around you.

You are supposed to love your body, you are supposed to love yourself, you are supposed to live with joy, you are supposed to have fun.

If you hadn't experienced what you don't want, how on earth would you know what you do want? What if they were simply lessons or even gifts, directing you towards bigger and better things? What if rather than life happening 'to' you, it was happening 'for' you? What if those doors that keep closing mean you simply need to turn around and find a window to climb out of instead - because there is something way better waiting beyond the walls you have built for yourself?

It might not be exactly how you want it right now, but sometimes the challenge we experience is necessary to prepare for the next wonderful level in life.

Stop defining yourself by the 'don't wants' and start using them as sign-posts to help guide you on your way. I truly believe it is impossible to be of service to anyone if we have not experienced their pain – how can we have empathy and walk by someone's side if we don't understand what they are going through? Sometimes pain is the very teacher you need to help you be the guide you were supposed to be for others. If you allow yourself to move through it rather than stay stuck in it, there is beautiful healing on the other side. The world needs you and the wisdom you have gleaned from your lessons.

From now on, let's look at the challenges as beautiful opportunities for growth that have helped you earn the stripes you can use to decorate your colourful wings. It is time to spread your wings wide and fly. Undo the shackles you have been holding yourself down with. Forgive yourself for all the self-judgement and criticism and recognise there is no such thing as failure, there is simply a lesson – always.

What I have learned so far in life is that being human is messy and it absolutely does not come without suffering. You will get things wrong but that does not make 'you' wrong or unloveable, you will experience challenges, things will feel hard – this is the beauty of being human. BUT (and it is a big but) you don't have to hold onto all of those things and define yourself by them. You can let go of the self-judgement and criticism and realise your own worth, your own light, and your own potential. You can start treating yourself with the loving kindness you are so very good at giving to everyone else.

This is what You Are Enough means. You don't have to prove yourself - and when you stop grasping and trying to prove your worth, everything becomes way easier and more enjoyable. You can simply have fun creating your very best life.

Beautiful goddess, life is waiting for you to live it.

Now is your time to start taking delicious steps in the full blazing glory of all that you are because you are truly a wonder. Life is simply waiting for you to realise it.

The only person you need to be is yourself. In fact, the more you shed the layers you've been dimming your light with and just allow your messy, beautiful, vulnerable, authentic, weird awesomeness to come forth, the more of you will shine. You are a joyful, complex, incredible and special individual - the world needs your colour because it is not the same as anyone else's.

Your soul asked to come into this life so that you could learn and grow. Every single person is here for a reason. It is your responsibility to move out of fear. It is your job to come home to yourself.

Healing is found in consciousness, self-forgiveness, in meeting all parts of ourselves, in appreciation and surrender, letting go and in love.

What you desire, desires you. It is yours if you allow it. You do not need to prove you are loveable or good enough. You simply are.

The work is to identify the beliefs you hold which do not align to what you desire.

Do you long to have a healthy body but hate, criticise and judge your own body and women who have a healthy body?

Do you long to have more abundance in your life but feel guilty for receiving money and judge people who do have abundance?

The energy you put out into the world is the very energy you will receive back.

It is essential to tune into the beliefs you hold and see how they align to what you really want.

It is your job to get out of your own way. So often we cling to what feels safe when a world of excitement, adventure, love, and joy awaits.

What do you need to let go of in order to allow in what you want?

What is the whispering of your soul truly hungry for?

It is my belief that when we are out of balance, over-critical of who we are, and lose the connection to our heart wisdom - which is so easy to do in this busy world - we use food or alcohol to numb the emptiness within.

You are enough. Be more of you. That is what the world needs. Not less.

Comparing, judging and holding yourself in shame is what dims your light. If I know one thing for sure, it's that the world needs your light. When a woman lights the torch within her, it spreads like wildfire to all of those around her and gives permission to everyone else to awaken their light too.

If you had any limiting beliefs, or fears of being judged or not good enough when you were little, you wouldn't be walking today, would you? You would have fallen over and given up a long time ago…but no, you got up and you tried again until you could walk and eventually run. At some point as we move into adulthood, we forget that learning new things takes practice, and instead we beat ourselves up for not being where someone else is, forgetting they have been practising for years. You have to be prepared to get it wrong in order to learn how to get it right.

You are the only person who limits you. The only person who is ever judging you is you. The Universe wants you to win. Yes – we all have different upbringings and experiences, but we are not defined by those. If we use those experiences to instead provide us with wisdom and insight we can learn how to love ourselves more. The work is always to give ourselves the validation we have been looking for externally.

Here is the piece you need to understand. Your worthiness is not defined or limited by any of the following:

- Having a beautiful, clean, tidy home
- Your ability to bake
- Whether you have children or not
- The clothes you wear
- The money you have
- The car you drive
- Your daily exercise intake
- How much you drank the night before
- How much TV you watch
- How often you meditate
- How happy your husband is in the bedroom
- Whether you have a partner at all
- How many friends you have
- How sociable you are or not

- The number on the scales
- The size of your home
- The job you have
- Whether you shouted at the kids yesterday
- What your hair looks like
- If you have been divorced (however many times!)
- What you said to someone last year, which you are still worrying about today

None of it. You are not defined by any of these things. These are external experiences and they do not define your worthiness. External things can change; you can change them. We get caught up in the stories of our mind, what society tells us we 'should' be, and lose sight of ourselves.

You wouldn't say 'I am a short bob' or 'I am a broken finger nail' and therefore it doesn't make sense to say 'I am overweight' or 'I am fat' either. Your body may be carrying some layers of additional energy because it is confused after years of restriction (don't worry – we will get to that too) but that is not WHO YOU ARE.

You are lovely. You are beautiful. You are strong. You are capable. You are wise. You are loveable. You can achieve whatever you put your mind to.

You were born with innate worthiness. You have always been the light within you. If you shine your light from that place of knowing, your life will unfold in remarkable ways and you can enjoy the ride!

You create your life experience from your thoughts, which create your belief system and guess what – your thoughts can change! Exciting!

As you go through this book, I ask you to put down your old ways of thinking and be open to the idea that you are actually an incredibly awesome woman who is ready to listen to the calling of her heart wisdom and show up for herself. And if you are thinking *that just isn't me*, then stick around...perhaps by the end of the book I might have managed to shift your thinking

One of my favourite quotes is by Marianne Williamson:

"Our deepest fear is not that we are inadequate. Our deepest fear is that we are powerful beyond measure. It is our light, not our darkness that most frightens us. We ask ourselves, 'Who am I to be brilliant, gorgeous, talented, fabulous?' Actually, who are you not to be? You are a child of God. Your playing small does not serve the world. There is nothing enlightened about shrinking so that other people won't feel insecure around you. We are all meant to shine, as children do. We were born to make manifest the glory of God that is within us. It's not just in some of us; it's in everyone. And as we let our own light shine, we unconsciously give other people permission to do the same. As we are liberated from our own fear, our presence automatically liberates others."

(And if you don't like the word God that is cool – simply replace it with Universe, Energy, Love…it doesn't matter. Whatever feels right for you.)

What you are searching for is already inside of you and it comes from YOU unlocking it. No one else can do it for you. Your healing starts with realising that you are enough and nothing outside of you will ever make you less or more. From there, you learn that you don't need to change anything to love who you are. Then you can start to nurture and nourish yourself in the way you have been longing for others to do for you for so long.

Where you focus your energy is what grows. This book is an invitation to focus your energy on the light within you. There is an old story about a Cherokee you may already be familiar with, but it is so important I want to share it with you again:

An old Cherokee is teaching his grandson about life. "A fight is going on inside me," he said to the boy. "It is a terrible fight and it is between two wolves. One is evil – he is anger, envy, sorrow, regret, greed, arrogance, self-pity, guilt, resentment, inferiority, lies, false pride, superiority, and ego.

He continued, "The other is good – he is joy, peace, love, hope, serenity, humility, kindness, benevolence, empathy, generosity, truth, compassion, and faith. The same fight is going on inside you – and inside every other person, too."

The grandson thought about it for a minute and then asked his grandfather, "Which wolf will win?"

The old Cherokee simply replied, "The one you feed."

I suspect you may have been focusing on the dark wolf, not the light – so let me guide you through how to shift that focus back to the beautiful one within you.

Throughout this book I am going to share affirmations to help you direct your thoughts and language towards the good wolf.

An affirmation is a statement that helps you change your energy in the moment by directing your thoughts. Remember, where you direct your energy is what grows, so you want to be directing your focus in a positive way.

The word affirmation comes from the Latin *affirmare*, originally meaning "to make steady, strengthen". You can use these to help you create new and loving ways of thinking and talking to yourself. Write them down in your journal, write them on post-it notes and stick them around your home, think them, say them out loud, or even shout them!

You can use one affirmation 50 times a day or write down 20 different ones every morning – what matters is that you're doing what you need to do to keep your energy high and your vibrations positive.

We can't choose how life happens to us, but we can choose how we respond. In fact, that's the only thing that we have the choice to do. You can reach for a thought that helps you feel better anytime you need to. You get to decide your own experience. What you put out in the world is what you receive in return.

It could be argued that the statements you put after I AM matter more than anything else you do. Your language matters on a very deep level. The statement 'I am' is how you identify and whatever you identify with, you will eventually become. It really is as simple as that. If you believe you are something because you have told yourself this enough times, that will become your reality. Be careful and gentle with your words and language.

As you develop your bank of affirmations, make sure they are not ones which feel too far away from where you are now. They need to make you feel good, not worse! Choose feel-good statements which don't feel like too far of a stretch for you to believe.

Affirmations

- I am enough

- I am loveable

- I let go of stories which are no longer serving my greater good

- I listen to my energy and direct my thoughts to ones which feel joyful.

Exercise 1

Take some time to answer the following questions in your journal:

- What has reading my story brought up for you about yours?

- What thoughts and beliefs are you ready to let go which are no longer of service to you?

- What makes you feel joyful?

- What frightens you the most?

- Where are you holding yourself back because of fear?

- What one thing could you do to love and accept yourself a little more deeply today?

Exercise 2

A practice that has been life-changing for me and which I regularly encourage women to practice in my coaching is self-celebration.

Hearing those words can be a bit toe-curling at first, but trust me!

If you are busy focusing on everything life is not, and you are constantly criticising yourself and your body - you ain't going to feel joyful, I know that for sure.

If life isn't feeling joyful - what do we do? We numb with food and we medicate with alcohol.

Our job is to get into a joyful state as much as possible. Even when life feels really hard, there is ALWAYS something to celebrate about you. You are your own heroine.

Life is not going to be better when you are thinner, have more money, have that dream house, or any of the other stories you have been telling yourself. The joy you seek is in this moment and that is the only place it is ever found. When you attach happiness to things outside of yourself, you are giving it a shelf life. If instead you seek joy in the moment for the very simple fact you are alive, your happiness cannot be taken away from you because it is not dependant on anything. From there, you will continue to create even more joy in your life. Joy is not what comes after you have achieved the next goal; that is upside down thinking. Joy is now, and you create and fulfil your desires from that place of joy.

Life is incredible right now and the only person who is going to help you realise that is you. From the foundation of incredible now, you can build your dreams.

Here is the practice...

Get out a journal and write 50 things you celebrate about yourself.

That might feel like a stretch right now but you can make a start and if it feels like a stretch then you have some work to do! It should be easy for you to do this - I know there are 1000s of things to celebrate about you, I am only asking for 50! Think about:

- How far have you come?

- What have you overcome?

- What have you achieved?

- When you look back over your life - how have you grown and changed?

- How do you serve others every day?

- How did you help someone?

- Who did you compliment?

Don't tell me there are not 50 things to celebrate about you - there are. Even if it is simply 'today I managed to get out of bed and get dressed'.

Get writing and notice the shift in your mood. Your true state is joyful; your job is to let that shine through!

So start celebrating!

Weight Loss Is Not the Goal

I suspect you are reading this book because of what it says on the cover, and that you want to finally break free from the perpetual cycle of dieting. I used to wake up and regret what I had eaten or drunk the day before, beat myself up, look in the mirror (if I could face it) and cringe. After Isaac came into the world, I remember wondering, *who am I?* I wasn't sure what to wear anymore – did becoming a Mum mean I needed to dress differently? Once, my favourite jeans ripped down the thigh because I had been squeezing myself into them for far too long and they no longer fit me. None of that mattered anyway because my self-loathing led me to hide my body under black, stretchy clothes, disguising my muffin top with baggy jumpers.

I tried every diet under the sun. I binged. I purged. I pinched. I hated. I starved. I restricted. I medicated with food and alcohol. All I could think about was food and when it would be a respectable time to have a drink – and then felt perpetual guilt when I did eat. If I shared food with friends or family, I compared the amount of food on my plate, what I had chosen to eat, and how fast I ate against everyone else.

I remember one particularly bad diet where I had been starving myself for days. I had also been taking packets of tablets that claimed to shrink fat cells. One day I was so hungry that, in a desperate moment, I pulled a cheesecake out of the bin and proceeded to eat the whole thing. How was this achieving my vision of happiness?! I have shared this story with so many women and when I see the relief that crosses their faces, it is incredibly healing for us both. You are not alone and your story is not shameful.

What if this focus on weight was the very cause of all the problems that are keeping you stuck?

I am going to let you in on a secret. I have absolutely no idea what I weigh. None at all. And I really, really don't care. I am the happiest I have ever been (and the slimmest – yes, it happened when I threw the scales away), I have the most energy I have ever had, I am the most confident I have ever been and I feel fantastic. Why would anything a number on the scales has to say be of any interest to me? And it shouldn't to you.

We must stop thinking that weight loss is the destination. Quite frankly – the goal of losing weight is boring, unimaginative, and depressing! It feeds directly into the patriarchal conditioning that runs so deeply through the blood of women and our ancestors. It does not honour the parts of yourself that are needing to be seen, heard and understood.

Weight loss is not your goal. Your goal is that thing you would LOVE to do, but have been putting off until the number on the scales says what you want it to. Your dreams and purpose are being sabotaged by your current belief that you are not worthy of achieving them until you reach a certain weight or look a certain way. There is not a single number on the scales that makes you more or less worthy.

Likewise, food is so much more than what you eat – it is how you nurture yourself in all aspects of your life. Ask yourself, "How do I feel full off my plate?" Primary food is how you fill up on LIFE. How do you express yourself? How do you honour all parts of who you are? Second-ary food is what you actually consume. When the balance between primary and secondary food is aligned and you feel full off your plate, your relationship with food will naturally come back into balance. We are going to get deeper into primary and secondary food later on in the section on pleasure. For now, simply start thinking about the concept of pleasure in life off your plate – how are you filling yourself up with fun, joy, laughter, connection, and purpose?

Let's move into a feminine and wise way of achieving what you desire. By creating a vision of what you want to achieve in your life (a purpose if you will) then weight and health becomes something that happens in service to that vision because you are having fun. When your body becomes a vehicle through which you experience life and you feel good in it, everything else becomes so much easier and more joyful. Let's make weight loss a happy accident because you are busy loving life!

When I was stuck in the dieting cycle, I had zero concept of what I wanted my future to look like. I was stuck in the day-to-day heaviness of beating myself up for what I looked like and what I ate. I also didn't realise I was hungry for more and that what I truly desired was my own love. I didn't have a clear long-term vision for the future. As it turns out, that was the very thing keeping me stuck. My sole purpose was to lose weight because I believed that would make me more worthy and ultimately happier.

Have you ever had a really solid vision that excites you about your future? Have you been waiting for life to begin after you lose weight? Do you believe you are only loveable when you weigh a specific number? How many times have you thought *I will do that when I am thinner?*

Right now, it might feel like getting to where you want to be is an impossible mountain to climb. Maybe you don't even know where to begin. Don't worry – let's break it down into steps to support you in moving forward towards your joy and wellbeing. I always think of it like a messy ball of string; we have to find the end and start unravelling it from there.

Your first step is no longer thinking about what you don't want but connecting with what you do. If you are anything like the way I was, then your approach has probably been working towards an ideal of what you *'no longer'* want. You *no longer* want to feel frumpy and tired, to cringe when you see a photo of yourself, to dread being seen naked, to hate the thought of clothes shopping and to allow the scales to determine your mood for the day. So here is the million-dollar question.

What DO you want?

What lights you up? What brings you joy? What makes you happy? What have you been putting off until the kids are older, the grandkids are older??

I regularly hear women say that they don't know who they are or what their purpose is, especially once their children have left home. Finding your purpose does not need to be anywhere near as scary as it first feels, and you don't need to find some huge, world changing idea to identify your purpose – you simply need to follow your bliss. By doing what you love to do, you will find yourself and your purpose will develop from there.

The question is, how much time do you allow yourself to do the things you love to do?

Life isn't waiting for you, so stop waiting for it to happen. It is happening right now. This is your life – today, this moment. This is a plea to you to live for today because this wonderful thing called life really is a beautiful thing when you choose to see it that way.

Your new way forward starts with stepping back, taking a look at the bigger picture and asking yourself what would really make you happy.

Having a vision of where you are going is the first step to achieving what you want. That is where many of us trip up, not allowing ourselves the pleasure of imagining.

What have you tricked yourself into believing you will be doing more of when you reach a certain weight? Do you think that you will be happier, change your job, set up that business, or experience a more fulfilled relationship?

You can have everything you want. You just need to stop putting it off and begin, and start living it right now. Remember, you are one of a kind. There is nobody else in the world like you, there never has been. This fact alone makes you a miracle. You are full of potential and possibility. Get creative with your vision. Allow yourself the luxury of creating. Play with ideas for your future. What thoughts truly fill your heart?!

Since infancy we have been taught to not think too big, and certainly not outside of the box! I am giving you the permission and space now to do just the opposite!

If you are not used to thinking about what you want in life, your head may start spinning with all the reasons you can't be, do or have the things you want. This is your internal dialogue popping up again and getting in the way of you living the life you deserve.

I really do get it. Remember, just six years ago I was in the depths of depression, eating cake out of a bin and drinking gin at 10.30am. Today I am sitting here writing this book after building a successful coaching business where I literally get to empower incredible women every day!

You too can achieve great things.

All great things begin with creating a vision of where you are going, and you do that by breaking it down. Use the exercise below to guide you through.

Affirmations

- My weight and worth are not connected
- I take steps towards things that feel blissful every day
- I am clear on my vision of the future
- It is safe for me to have desires
- I am worthy of creating my dream life
- It is safe for me to enjoy food

Exercise

What do you want to create in your life?

Below I share with you some sections you can use to chunk your life into manageable pieces. Similar to a wheel of life, which you might well have come across before, this will help you think about what needs your attention and what you really want.

Take time to go through each life area and get clear on what you would like to see happening in the next month, next six months, the next year and the next five years:

- My health and wellbeing

- My relationship with myself

- My intimate relationship

- My family

- My friends

- My career

- My joy

- My finances

Once you have defined what you want and written it down, the next step is to explore WHAT you need to do in order to achieve that. What is the first little step you need to take? I suggest starting each day by asking yourself what action you need to take today to move you forward towards your goal.

Focus on what you do want, not what you don't want. Your brain is designed to move away from pain and towards pleasure. Get excited about the positive future outcomes you would like to move towards.

For example, move from the notion of 'I want to lose 10lbs' to 'I want to jump out of bed in the morning with vitality and energy, confidently put my jeans on without even thinking about it and freely go wild swimming naked in the sea'. The energy around these statements is different – can you feel it? One feels heavy and one feels exciting!

The question moving forward is not 'what do you want to weigh?' but 'what extraordinary things do you want to experience in your life?'

Get excited about where you are going!

Nudging Out of Comfort

It is normal to feel overwhelmed when you first start making changes in your life. It can feel like there are so many things to tackle. Know that you don't have to make huge, monumental shifts to transform your life. In fact, the more subtle ones practised regularly will have a much bigger impact.

Start with one.

One step forward.

One cup of water.

One yoga class.

One good night's sleep.

One word in your journal.

One old contact deleted.

One.

It starts there.

Change takes place when we follow the energy of feeling good every day rather than waiting to feel good until you have achieved everything you desire.

If you focus on the big changes you want to make it is likely you will find yourself stuck in overwhelm and that often leads to fruitless comparison. Simply hitting a golf ball with a 2-millimetre difference on impact changes the trajectory enormously when it hits the fairway. Incremental mini shifts are your way forward – your job is to chunk it down and make it manageable. That is why I love the wheel of life – choose one aspect which you would like to work on for a month and focus solely on that. Almost every time I work with a woman, she says, "If I focus on my health and physical wellbeing and my relationship with myself – everything else will fall into place." I suspect that goes for you, too.

The trick is to then gently nudge yourself out of comfort a little bit every day.

Consistency is key. Change is a constant practice, not an all or nothing approach. Over time your comfort zone expands and expands until all of a sudden you are living an unrecognizable life.

We are designed as humans to stay in our comfort zone. It is what has made us so successful from an evolutionary standpoint. But your comfort zone isn't serving you anymore. It is time to move into your stretch zone, the happy place between boredom and panic. The place where you grow and learn and find joy in life because you are moving one step at a time towards your goals and desires.

Staying stuck in your comfort zone is one of the biggest reasons you lean on food for comfort and to fill you up. In order to feel alive you must have purpose. You have to feel excited about life. If everything has become too boring or mundane; if you follow the same route to work every day, do a job which is not fulfilling, or perhaps feel life has become a safe and unadventurous routine, of course you will look for comfort. The truth of you is joyful and playful, and she loves adventure and fun.

You don't need to be taking huge and drastic action, but I do suggest you gently nudge yourself out of your comfort zone a little every day. Do things that are different. Try new things. Smile at a stranger, give someone a compliment, wear colour, read instead of watch TV, go for dinner by yourself. Take a different route to work. Do things that feel good, exciting and fun!

Life expands outside of your comfort zone. It is OK to live in discomfort and in fact that is where you grow. If my life is feeling uncomfortable, I have trained myself to think, *yay – there is some growing coming my way. What is the Universe giving me that I am ready to learn?* It is not always pleasant, yet one of the most life-changing revelations for me has been that the more OK I get with being uncomfortable, the more I grow and the more enjoyable life becomes.

For a caterpillar to become a butterfly it must first become a chrysalis. During this transition it becomes liquid and the only part of it which stays the same is its eyes. It is safe for you to lose yourself to find your way home; you might just need to do that to be able to spread your beautiful wings. The question is, where are you keeping yourself stuck so that you feel safe and where is this making you unhappy? When we are unhappy, we look for comfort in things which are not necessarily serving us. We say "I can't break this pattern" when in fact we are the ones who are creating it. Part of your healing is realising you are the creator of your own reality and have 100% responsibility for your choices.

When we disconnect our worth from external success (whatever we deem success to be) and allow ourselves to be excited about the journey towards where we are going – life becomes very different indeed. Celebrating yourself and the little wins every day creates new neural pathways in your mind so that new habits become easier and easier. Looking back and reflecting on how far you have come is an extremely important and powerful practice because it gives you perspective. Rather than seeking to find fault in what you have not yet achieved, shift your focus to what is wonderful about what you have done.

Affirmations

- It is safe for me to love myself

- It is safe for me to celebrate all that I am

- It is safe for me to move forward out of my comfort zone and try new things

Exercise

Draw two circles. The first one represents your comfort zone. This zone might feel like a security blanket but really, being here all the time is simply not serving you – it is time to step out and shine your Goddess Light.

Write down all the ways you are staying in your comfort zone right now. What actions, conversations or steps are you not taking for fear of discomfort?

The second circle is your stretch zone. This is the zone from which you want to live your life, gently moving yourself outside of your zone of comfort, learning and growing and taking new steps into the unknown a little more each day. One step at a time is enough. It is small steps and actions taken consistently which build up to great change over time.

What next steps do you need to take to move forward? Break the big scary changes into bite-sized, manageable actions. Remember – you will not feel comfortable taking these steps. You are primed for safety. Uncomfortable DOES NOT mean don't do it – it means you are in a zone of growth.

Your comfort zone will expand as you take brave steps outside of it and allow your world to grow in ways beyond your wildest expectations.

What action steps can you take that feel stretchy to move you towards your goals? Make some notes in your journal about actions you can take to nudge you out of comfort. You will probably find these little nudges align with the goals you set out in the previous section.

Glow From Within

You might have heard the saying 'love the skin you are in' before but I don't think that goes far enough. I think we all need to go even deeper than that. This is about truly loving yourself at your core. As I started to work with women and help them move into their true power, I realised I was going to need to do some pretty deep work myself. How could I help if I wasn't coming from a place of authenticity or experience?

One morning, as I was busy covering myself in make-up, judging and criticising how I looked at every step, a little voice inside piped up and said, "Glow from within." It really struck a chord with me and has stayed with me ever since.

Glow from within.

Huh. Had I ever trusted my body to glow? Had I ever thought about the nutrients I was putting into it? Had I ever supported it and helped it thrive in the way I was so desperately looking for? I had never considered that my body is amazing and will do everything I want it to if I just look after it.

What if we can all glow, and that is in fact what human bodies do when we nurture them? If I wanted to glow, look healthy, and lose weight, how on earth could I expect that to happen if I wasn't taking care of myself? At that time, I was drinking at least a bottle of wine a night, fighting a constant battle with my body. I was poisoning myself every day and criticising it when it didn't look how I wanted it to. Imagine pouring gin and sugar into the soil of your favourite pot plant every day and then criticising it when it inevitably gets sick! Yet I realised that was what I had been doing to myself since I was a teenager. It was my mindset that was going to need to shift, not my body.

One big hangup I would need to move past was around the colour of my skin. I am one quarter Scottish, one quarter Welsh, and half English. As skin colour goes – you aren't going to get much fairer than that. I do not tan. Ever. I have two shades: pink and white! And since my teenage years, I believed this was deeply unattractive. In the 90s it was trendy to be tanned and that was just not me.

So I hid. I covered every part of my body behind fake tan or clothings. I never wore shorts, and if I wore skirts, I wore tights underneath. Fake tan wasn't much better; it just resulted in me turning orange, sporting stained fingernails, smelling of biscuits, and brown bed sheets to boot – it really wasn't a great look! But I believed I was only attractive when I was covered or fake-tanned, so no-one ever saw me otherwise. It became a problem because it meant I needed to spend hours tanning before I could do anything else.

There was a time in my 20s when I was travelling in Thailand and I was invited out on a boat for the day – it would have been amazing. But I turned it down. Why? Because I was terrified of being seen without a tan, and it happened to need redoing on this particular day. (Fake tan is really hard to get hold of on Thai islands because everyone wants to be pale – how insane is that? We all want something different in order to feel we are enough.) I stayed in my Thai bungalow all day until the sun went down and it was dark enough for me to go out without people seeing the colour of my skin.

I have missed out on many opportunities as a result of saying no simply because I was worried about not being good enough. I hid every part of myself. That belief got deeper and more powerful. I hid my hands by tucking them into my sleeves – I believed even my hands were ugly. As I am sitting here writing on my laptop, I look down at my hands and wonder how I could have ever thought that. Look at what they are doing for me now! I get to share this with you today because of them – what a gift and opportunity.

So when this voice said "Glow from within" I knew what I needed to do, or at least where I needed to start. I decided I would walk into town without fake tan on my arms wearing a vest top. I was TERRIFIED. It took so much courage to step out of my front door and when I did, I ran straight back inside again. But I KNEW I needed to do this so I took a deep breath and I stepped back outside, closed the front door and started walking.

I was so nervous. I felt the whole world would judge me for being so ugly. What I now know is that my fear was of not being accepted. At a survival level, to not be accepted by society means death. Of course I wasn't going to die, but I carried a belief that to be loveable I had to look a certain way, and to challenge that was a huge step. "Here I am world, in my own version of me and I don't need your acceptance."

I walked into town and, shock horror, bumped into someone I knew. OH MY GOD. But guess what? They didn't mention a thing and in fact, they didn't even notice. It simply wasn't a big deal.

I went home. Nothing happened. The world didn't end. I obviously didn't die.

It led me to think – the only person whose opinion matters is my own. If I can learn to love this body I live in, then that is enough.

My job was to love myself and learn to love this pale skin I live in. It makes me who I am. Whilst I might not look like a Californian beach babe, I am me and that is enough. No one except me actually cares.

The love I was looking for comes from me, and only me.

Affirmations

- I love my body and my body loves me

- My body wants to glow with health and vitality

- I take time to nourish my body with all that it needs in thought and action

Exercise

- Have a think and/or journal about your relationship with your body.

- What language do you use in relation to your body?

- If your body was a person, how would it feel about being in a relationship with you?

- How many times a day do you think negatively about your body compared to how many times you think positively?

- What steps can you take to shift towards kind and loving language about your body?

- What does your body need to feel better?

- How does your body show up for you every day?

- What would celebrating your body look and feel like to you?

Your Hungry Divinity

Women obsess over their weight and size, not because we are shallow, but because every day we're told our worth hinges on our looks. We live in a culture where it's normal to judge an actress based on her body size and the supermarket shelves are full of magazines that encourage this kind of discussion.

In truth, dieting is a distraction from the real and authentic work women need to do to move away from this deep social conditioning.

At the Peace Conference in Canada in 2009, the Dalai Lama said, "The world will be saved by the Western Woman."

What has this got to do with weight loss, I hear you ask? Let me explain.

There is still a part of you which needs to be deeply understood. Who is desperate to be heard, to be seen, expressed, and to be free. She is the wild part of you, the woman inside of you who has been caged and told what it is to be a woman. Told what to say, what to wear, how to look.

There is a goddess within you. Your Divine Feminine. Soul. Intuition. Knowing. The Loving Voice within you. Whatever name you want to give her, she is the reason why you have picked up this book and she is what will lead you to the healing you seek.

I bet you have read loads of books about what to eat and how to be healthy. If they had the answers, why are you here?

Your body was born to glow with vitality, be filled with energy, and find a normal weight – all she asks is for you to stop restricting and start nourishing her with the food you eat and the words you speak to her.

Shift your focus to appreciating your beautiful body as she is now. You won't take good care of something you hate. Instead of depriving your body, think about nourishing it so you can accomplish all the amazing things you are capable of.

Your body is amazing! Slow down and listen to her, build a relationship with her, talk to her, ask her what it needs. She is longing for you to love her.

You were born whole. We all are. Whether you are male or female, you are equal parts masculine and feminine energy. Masculine energy is goal oriented, thinking with logic, and taking action. The patriarchal world we live in is entrenched in the masculine, and because we have been taught to lean so heavily into the masculine elements the equally powerful and important feminine elements such as pleasure, intuition, listening, and sensuality get over-looked or even judged and criticised. I have worked with so many women who think that because they can't logi-cally explain what they feel intuitively, what they have to say is not valid. I struggled with this for years too. I felt silenced at the dinner table or in meetings, embarrassed to say what I was thinking because it was coming from a place of heart feeling rather than brain logic. If it doesn't feel right, you can trust that. You can trust your intuition - she is powerful.

Your not being smart or clever is so far from the truth and is simply what patriarchal conditioning wants you to believe. Millions of women have been murdered over the years for being intuitive (I was shocked to learn that num-ber too!), burned, drowned and murdered for the wisdom they possessed. That fear has been carried down through generations of women. Because we have been taught that a true and real part of ourselves is not valid, that we are only worthy because of how we look or if we take mascu-line action, we create beliefs that we are not good enough.

In order to create wellbeing in your life, you need to find balance in both masculine and feminine energies. Your femininity is not weak, she is powerful. Think about how many people struggle to trust their intuition. It shows how out of balance we are. If we are too much in our masculine or we are ignoring our feminine (this applies to both men and women) then this can spill over into unhealthy masculine and feminine energies. (Towards the end of this section, I have outlined how both are expressed in behaviours, to help you identify where you might want more balance.)

There is absolutely nothing wrong with masculine energy, yet if you are in it all of the time, you are dishonouring the divine feminine who also sits within you. Your feminine wisdom is hungry to be heard, seen, and celebrated. She is expressed through nurturing, abundance, sensuality, and wisdom. She connects to nature, she stops to connect with her breath, notice the beauty around her, she trusts her intuition, and she takes time to smell the roses. She is glorious and powerful.

A huge part of the work in healing our relationship with our bodies and food is seeing through the years and layers of patriarchal conditioning and reconnecting to the truth.

Truth: your body is beautiful.

Truth: there isn't a number on the scales which makes you more worthy.

Truth: you came here for a reason. You are inherently worthy and you are needed.

Truth: your healing will heal others

If you are ready to tear down and burn the years of conditioning and shame connected to being a woman then you are in the right place, sister.

At this point, you might feel deeply disconnected from yourself. You might not have ever known another version of you existed. You might have so many voices in your head you have no idea which one to listen to. I promise she IS in there – within you. You haven't managed to get this eating thing under control yet because you have been fed so much nonsense about dieting and you are disconnected from the truth of who you are. Love yourself first and food falls into place. That is the real way forward. Your healing starts with turning everything you have been taught on its head.

Dieting is BS. It feeds directly into the deep shame that keeps women churning through the same cycle for their whole lives. Just imagine what you could do if you weren't spending a huge proportion of your time worrying about what you look like!

Society has taken a masculine approach to health and weight loss, which is why so many people are stuck in constant cycles of dieting, eating, guilt, and shame. Women have been taught that to be enough they must look a certain way. Every part of that message is dishonouring your femininity. The truth is, when you slow down, listen to your body, and your intuition, you will learn how to nurture and nourish her with all that she needs. From there, your health and perfect weight will appear as if by magic. Your body wants you to be well and healthy. You need to stop being at war with it and with yourself. Get out of your head and move into your heart.

The best and most beautiful things in the world, cannot be seen or even touched - they must be felt with the heart. The way people feel in your presence is your gift to the world so start there. Start with how it feels for you to be in your heart.

How are you honouring the Divine Feminine with you? Take time to sit and listen to your needs without the distraction of your phone. Just doing that might be deeply uncomfortable for you to begin with – that is OK.

How much time have you made for your own pleasure in the last week?

The feminine is found in being, not doing; experiencing pleasure and the joy of being alive instead of getting somewhere.

Pleasure might look like:

- Slowing down, connecting with your breath, noticing the joy around you

- Leaving the never-ending to-do list and doing something you enjoy instead

- Massage and touch

- Making love

- Practising gratitude

- A bath without your phone

- Candles and sensual music

- Reading for pleasure

- Walking in nature

- Moving your body (not to burn calories, but because it feels good)

- Cooking yourself a beautiful meal and tasting each bite

There Is No Guilt In Pleasure

You connect to your Divine Feminine through experiencing pleasure in your body. Through self-care, touch, connection, breath, massage, bathing, sexual pleasure, soft music, candles, relaxing, dance, movement, down-time.

What do those words make you feel? Is the word 'pleasure' triggering for you? These might be uncomfortable questions but are a really important part of your healing:

- Do you feel guilty if you slow down or take time for yourself?

- How often do you think you must get your to-do list done rather than take time for self-care?

- Do you receive pleasure sexually or do you ensure your partner is always satisfied and ignore your own needs?

- Do you get your hair or nails done not for your pleasure but in order to look a certain way?

When we are triggered it is a calling to look within. It is a sign there's something to be learned. Instead of shrinking away from things that make you feel uncomfortable, move towards them. If a word makes you cringe or gasp, from now on, ask why.

Why have we put the words 'guilty' and 'pleasure' together? Why is pleasure guilty?

We have been so deeply conditioned to believe that as women, we are 'bad' for receiving pleasure or being in our feminine. To be successful in life, to be a good girl, and to be loved - you must give, you must do, you must be busy. You must prove your worth through how you look and how you serve. We are given play kitchens and taught we are good girls for serving everyone tea! When did anyone ever tell you as a child to put yourself first or ask what you need?

We tend to feel guilt when we do things for ourselves – we have always been taught to do things for others. But self-care and pleasure are not selfish. When you are good, everyone else is better. They get you from your full cup, not what's left after you have taken care of everyone else.

It has been ingrained in many of us that receiving pleasure is neither safe nor acceptable. From the precious and impressionable time when we first move into womanhood and onwards, our bodies are judged. Too tall, too thin, too fat... "It is just puppy fat, dear." "You are big boned." "You need to go on a diet." The list is endless. It is not uncommon for our male caregivers to no longer know how to talk to us when we become women. We absorb the message that becoming a woman means losing the love of a safe man. I remember my girlfriends taunting me when I started my period at 12! Why? These were my friends. But it was not their fault – it is part of the systemic conditioning that being a woman is shameful.

Pleasure is bad, dirty, slutty, promiscuous...

Of course, none of this is true. Pleasure is in fact essential to our wellbeing. But we have been so deeply conditioned over the centuries that shame runs deep through our veins. The shame of celebrating your body, loving who you are, and celebrating yourself.

If you feel guilt about receiving pleasure through any form of self-care at all, where is the one last place you can connect with the pleasure your soul is hungry for? You guessed it...through food.

Feeding Your Soul

What is it about food that makes it feel so hard? Why do I keep eating? Why, when I lose weight, do I put it all back on again? I am a smart, capable woman – why does this feel like the one thing I can't succeed at? Is eating less really that hard?

The truth is this. You have been sleepwalking through a patriarchal world, conditioned by society and generations of ancestors to believe that pleasure and self-care are not important and in fact, are something to be frowned upon.

Your relationship with food runs so much deeper than you have been led to believe. If you hold beliefs about receiving pleasure and the full expression of your femininity being unsafe and unloveable; about your worth being defined by busyness and external achievement, then of course you are going to use food to find that little bit of pleasure in your life. Of course you are going to try and fill that gaping hole with something that is socially acceptable.

- Do you feel guilt when you eat?

- Do you find it difficult to receive pleasure?

- Do you push away a compliment when you receive one?

- Do you find it hard to ask for help?

- Do you feel vulnerability is a weakness?

All of these feelings are wrapped up in shame with a big bow on top. Shame keeps us quiet. We push those feelings down and make sure no-one will ever know about them because then they might find out we are not good enough. What do we do when we push our feelings down? You guessed it again – we eat.

Do you eat in secret? I used to. I would drive to a petrol station and buy crisps, sandwiches, and chocolate bars, eat them quickly before I got to where I was going, and then hide the evidence! I don't know who I was kidding. Who was I hiding from? Myself? The reason you eat in secret is because you are truly hungry in your body and your soul, and the only way you believe you can receive that nurturing and nourishing is through food.

Society teaches us that pleasure is found in buying and having more, but that just leads to feeling more empty. Your soul is hungry for pleasure and food provides that, but you need it in so many other ways.

Remember that primary food has nothing to do with what you eat; rather it's about how you receive pleasure and joy in your life through sources other than food. Secondary food is what you eat. Food is the one socially acceptable pleasure for most women, and it's time to reclaim all the other forms of pleasure that perhaps you have been denying yourself. If I notice my balance is leaning towards food then I ask myself where I have let things slip. Perhaps you might find this a helpful concept too.

Split your life into areas – nourishment off your plate and nourishment on your plate. It makes sense that you would look for pleasure in an area of your life where you need it, and if you are not experiencing joy in any other place than food – what are you going to do?

It is time to bring back the simple pleasure of joy and take action to fill up your primary food cup. What you have been searching for in food is not found in food (or indeed alcohol) - but you already know that! It is found in what lights you up in life.

Take a moment to think about where you feel the most alive. In your career? In your intimate relationship? In your community? In your home environment? With your family and friends?

What lights you up? What sets your world on fire? What gives you hope?

Has fear stopped you from taking steps towards what you want in your life? Has life just got a little bit too small for your expansive heart?

How much joy and pleasure do you experience on a daily basis? Has life become a little bit too serious - filled with endless to-do lists or serving everyone apart from yourself?

What has led to things being that way? More importantly, what needs to change in order for that to be different?

How do you have fun and how much of it are you having?

When did you last belly laugh until you cried?

What fills you up with joy?

How do you need to start nourishing your hunger without food?

Your head might well answer "I don't know" to these questions but you do know. Your heart knows. This book is not for your head, it is for your hungry heart.

A practice I find really powerful if I am struggling to find an answer is asking myself the question before I go to sleep. Nine times out of 10, I wake up with the answer. Give it a go.

Resting and Rebalancing

If you keep putting back on the weight you have lost, it is because you are carrying a subconscious narrative that pulls you back into your old pattern. It is important to achieve a goal by aligning with it energetically, not forcing yourself to get there because you believe you should. If you don't feel worthy of anything that you create in your life, it is not possible to maintain it because your energy is not aligned to it.

Patriarchy says we should be a certain way to be good enough. Remember, you do not need to lose weight to be loveable or socially acceptable. You already are those things. You already live in a beautiful body – she will glow for you when you love her now, not on a conditional basis. If instead you slow down and nurture all that you are with love, you will learn to listen to your intuition and wisdom. From that place you will be able to create a healthy relationship with food and if you desire weight loss it will become a happy accident instead of a battle.

Society leans heavily on the masculine side of being human. It has taught us that it is weak to be in our feminine and that is simply not true. What is truly powerful is an equal balance of feminine and masculine energy, and that is where healing lies.

Heck, women even exercise from the masculine, with the goal to burn calories and be thin. What would it be like to simply move because it feels good and trust your body will find health when you love it, slow down, and relax? Your body loves to move to release energy and keep your cells vital, you don't have to smash your body to burn calories.

There is a story about an artist who was lying down. Someone came up to him and said, "You are resting" and he replied, "No, I am working." When he was painting, someone came up to him and said, "You are working" and he replied, "No, I am resting." Knowing who you are does not come from busyness, it comes through connection to yourself and following your bliss.

Rest allows you to be more productive. Fortifying your cup of energy through rest will reinvigorate you, and true, grounded confidence will shine from your pores because you know who you are and where you are going.

It is safe for you to rest, it is safe for you to slow down, it is safe for you to stop and listen.

By the way, rest is not completing your to-do list, or doing your chores because they don't take much thinking. It is not cleaning the house, doing the laundry, or tidying the kitchen. Rest is being. It is doing nothing for pleasure; reading, drawing, creating, moving, stillness, being in nature.

There is no guilt or shame in rest, slowing down, and listening. In fact, these are all necessary for you to reconnect with the truth of who you are. You will not reach your full potential or find health and wellbeing in constant doing and pushing. When you start to see rest, pleasure, sensuality, and slowing down as the path back to the truth of who you are – you will be able to listen to your heart's beautiful wisdom.

Along the way, you may notice some fears or resistance pop up. After all, it is weak to be girly. It means you need to wear pink, be blonde (nothing wrong with being blonde by the way – I am with a little help!) and have long nails. Right?

NO. That is what patriarchal conditioning has done – led us to believe that being in our feminine is not strong. Being in your feminine is incredibly powerful. She uses her intuition. She is a powerful knowing coming from a place of grounded authenticity. She expresses the truth of who she is. She sets boundaries with love. She likes movement, not to burn calories or achieve a certain body shape, but to celebrate her body as it is.

Like water, she is a force of nature; she can move mountains and equally flow gently and softly. She is calm, soothing, peaceful, beautiful, as well as stormy, wild, and dangerous. She rests and she moves. She gives life, but you must respect her power. Just like Bruce Lee said: "Be like water."

Don't ignore the beautiful force within you because you are worried about creating a storm or what others might think of you. It is time to stop apologising and start allowing yourself to be expressed. Honouring your femininity is an essential part of your healing.

The Divine Feminine is within all of us. When we live too much in the external world and ignore our feminine needs, we feel unheard, fearful, a victim to our circumstances. We believe we are powerless. This is never the truth. We need to tune into the truth of who we are and come home to ourselves.

An empowered woman lights up all the women around her, like a candle being passed forward. Empowered women empower other women. If you want to change the world, start by changing yourself.

This is an invitation to look within and create space for self-enquiry. Make a commitment to get to know yourself. Your soul is hungry for empowerment and wholeness. What you are seeking is your own attention, love, and acceptance.

You are found in quiet reflection. In order to truly heal, you must slow down and meet all the parts of who you are. When you do this without judgement, you can fully love and embrace yourself.

It's important to know that both masculine and feminine energies have an unhealthy, wounded aspect and a healthy, divine aspect. The wounded part comes from ego, a place of fear and darkness - and always leads to pain.

Have a look at these healthy and unhealthy masculine and feminine traits and reflect on which ones you would like more or less of:

- **Healthy Feminine**: Grounded, compassionate, asks for what she needs, vulnerable, is comfortable in her body, uses wisdom and intuition, playful, joyful, authentic, creates and births, connects and brings people together in community, attuned to energy.

- **Unhealthy Feminine**: Insecure, critical, needy, blows up because her needs are not met, fears loss, can be manipulative, chases love or is over attached to people to fulfil her needs, takes care of others before herself, self-sacrificing, and does not honour or connect to her internal wisdom.

- **Healthy Masculine**: Creates safety, observes without judgement, is present, seeks stillness and silence, accepts things come to an end, disciplined, has mentors and serves others, is committed to truth and growth, action comes from slowing down and connecting.

- **Unhealthy Masculine**: Competitive, focused on success, cold and distant, afraid of failure, has to be right, tries to fix everything, runs away from love, does not think about others, reactive, constantly pushing forward.

Read through these and make a note of things you would like to work on.

Remember, we all hold both masculine and feminine traits. If we lean too much toward one of the other, we tend to fall into an unhealthy balance. Use this exercise to identify what you want to do more of and less of. It is time to heal by moving into the healthy parts of yourself, giving yourself permission to express who you are to the world!

Affirmations

- It is safe for me to receive pleasure

- It is safe for me to take time to rest

- I celebrate my femininity

- I tune into the feminine knowing within me

- I trust my intuition and wisdom

- It is safe for me to ask for what I need

Exercise

It is safe for me to receive pleasure in ways other than food.

What does this affirmation bring up for you? Read it and sink into your body – do you experience any energetic shifts, any fear in your throat, prickles of anxiety, or butterflies in your tummy?

Simply be interested without judgement. If this statement creates an energetic response in your body or mind, it is an indication that your nervous system holds beliefs that were created to protect you and keep you safe.

What beliefs do you think are related to this statement for you and where do you think they came from?

Have a think about how you feel about pleasure and receiving.

What did you experience during your first or early sexual experiences? Did you feel safe and loved?

Have you been taught that it is safe to be vulnerable and to receive pleasure or is there a deep-seated self-preservation within you when it comes to these things?

Make time and space to build a relationship with yourself, to listen to your needs and desires. It doesn't have to be huge, drastic action; in fact, it is better if it is not.

Simply start your days by asking yourself these questions:

- What do I need to be joyful today?

- What beliefs do I hold which make me feel uncomfortable with experiencing pleasure and what am I ready to believe instead?

- What one thing could I do to take me out of my comfort zone and into my excitement zone?

Are Your Stories Keeping You Stuck?

As I mentioned back in the introduction, there was a time when I went to buy nappies and my card got declined. I didn't have enough money to buy my son what he needed. It was the most ashamed I have ever felt.

I had a relatively good job at the time. I should have had enough money to buy him what he needed but instead I was throwing money away on wasteful things because I didn't believe I was worthy enough to take care of myself in any form – even financially. Not being able to buy my son what he needed served me in a way because it fed even more deeply into my story of being stuck. *See – look how hard this is, I can't even buy nappies.*

I was making my own life harder, creating challenges because at a subconscious level I didn't believe I was good enough. I didn't know this at the time, but now I see I was fully responsible for what I created. To truly heal, we have to get honest about why the pattern we are so keen to let go of at a logical level is actually serving us at a sub-conscious level.

The need for safety is what drives us all. Sometimes the fear of moving outside of what we know, even if what we know is not making us happy, feels incredibly hard because from a survival perspective, new is dangerous.

According to American psychiatrist and psychologist, Milton Erickson, "all problems were once our solutions". In effect, the things that feel like they are keeping us stuck are the very things we created at some point to keep us safe. I regularly see women unconsciously holding onto weight because they do not feel safe in the world. If a woman has received unwanted sexual attention, it makes sense that her subconscious would create a pattern to hold her at a heavier weight to keep her safe. The solution is therefore finding a new way of creating safety through love instead of fear.

As you are becoming aware, this book is ultimately about your relationship with yourself – or more importantly, it is about self-love. Above all, loving yourself is the most important thing you can do. Every part of your wellbeing and joy comes from your own self-acceptance. As Einstein said, everything is energy, and the life you experience comes from the energy you put out into the world. It is impossible for you not to get back what you put out. The work you do within will shine brightly into the experience you receive back on your journey.

Weight loss doesn't come from a focus on weight loss. Your relationship with food is merely the symptom, not the cause. Beneath every single behaviour is a feeling and if you allow yourself to feel the feeling, explore it and recognise what it really needs, then you can identify the cause.

- How often do you think about what you really need?

- How often do you offer loving kindness to yourself?

- How often do you slow down and take time for you?

If you keep going and keep being busy, ignoring and dishonouring your needs, you will never hear the voice guiding you. You always have an answer, and you do know the next step – the real question is, have you slowed down enough to listen to yourself?

I once coached a lady who felt very stuck, and was finding it difficult to understand why she couldn't make progress in the way she desired. If she did, she sabotaged her success and went back to square one.

One day, I asked, "What are you celebrating about yourself today?" She responded, "I am celebrating that I am able to offer love to those who are less fortunate than me." Interesting. I then asked, "Do only people who are less fortunate than you deserve love?" She looked at me, astonished. "I have always thought only people who suffer deserve to be loved! I was sick as a child and my brother always did better at school than me, so I got attention from my parents through my sickness." Wow – this was a lightbulb moment for her. She realised she had been holding herself back because she believed if she got to where she wanted to be, she would no longer be worthy of receiving love. This was her way of loving and protecting herself. Through this realisation, she was able to let that pattern go and move forward to finally achieve what she wanted.

I don't believe in linear learning, so although she felt she wasn't making progress, she always was. There is great learning in everything we experience. Sometimes we have to let go of our attachment to how we want it to be and on the time-scale we want. In order to achieve what we desire, we need to get out of our own way.

The energy you put out is the energy you get back. If at your core, you do not believe you are worthy or loveable but you are externally trying to prove yourself, you will keep coming back to where you feel stuck. You have to do the inner work. You have to get the internal aligned with the external. You have to realise how worthy you truly are.

Within each of us is an ego and authentic self. The word ego is often misunderstood. Your ego is your sense of self-preservation and is actually coming from a need for love and safety. People might be seen to be in their ego when really, they are hiding their fear. Perhaps they feel ashamed or that they won't be accepted if they are vulnerable, so they build a wall to protect themselves. Ego is demonstrated through a range of behaviours, from bravado to limiting beliefs. Ego is what keeps you out of alignment with who you truly are. Ego creates patterns in your subconscious to keep you safe.

When you were born you were a blank canvas and as you grew, you watched everyone around you so that you could figure out how to survive in this world. Your physiology is designed to soak everything up like a sponge. Your mind created patterns and behaviours to ensure you were accepted, loveable, and ultimately remain alive. As a child, if you are loved you are safe. Between the ages of one and 10, our sole need is to be loved and feel we are enough.

I don't believe anyone comes through childhood unscathed. There is not a single person on this planet who has not experienced some degree of trauma in their lives. Trauma doesn't have to be a big disastrous event. It can be something as simple as a new sibling coming along and your parents not being as available to you, or a teacher shaming you, making you feel stupid.

It is actually small and consistent trauma that does more damage in many cases. As children, we make meaning out of those experiences and hard wire them into our belief system to protect us. That one experience can be carried through the rest of our lives and we then consistently look for evidence to prove that it is true.

You might have had the most outwardly perfect childhood, but if you didn't feel loveable as a child or you were raised by emotionally unavailable parents or caregivers, this creates two things:

1. Beliefs that you are not good enough or not worthy. If it is not the fault of the adult (and a child would

never think that it was) it must be your fault. (Of course, this isn't the case – but that is how a child interprets it.)

2. A disconnection from yourself. How can you trust and love who you are if you feel so deeply unloveable? From there, deep beliefs about lack of self-worth are created and that results in struggles with confidence and low self-esteem.

Our subconscious then creates patterns of safety. *If you stay small, unseen or don't speak up you are safe. Don't be vulnerable and show your emotions – it is weak. Don't let people in, they will hurt you. If you truly let someone in, they will see who you really are and leave you. Don't choose a good guy because you don't deserve to be treated well. Only when you weigh a certain amount are you loveable. Don't be greedy. Don't have needs. Please other people so that they like you. Put other people's needs before your own and then you will be enough. Clear your plate, there are starving children in the world.*

It embeds them into the brain so we don't have to remember them. They become our go-tos, just like when you instinctively try to turn on a light switch even though you know there is a power cut on, or you try and put your foot on the brake even though you are in the passenger's seat. You have copied behaviours from the people around you or created patterns to ensure an experience that hurt or scared you doesn't happen again.

I think of the ego like your loving safety lock. It is designed to keep you safe and protected but it also keeps you small. Let's face it, some of the stories it has made up to keep you safe are downright unkind and absolutely untrue. The problem is, you might have been stuck in these stories for so long that you actually believe them. Maybe you didn't even know there was another part of you that is your truth. She is the loving, nurturing part of you and it is time for you to offer yourself the same kindness and grace you dutifully dole out to everyone else. I often say to my clients, if you spoke to a little girl the way you speak to yourself every day of your life, how happy would she be? And they are always horrified. They say, "I would never do that. That would be awful."

But that is what you do to yourself every day.

Yes, your subconscious *thinks* it is keeping you safe and protecting you by whispering in your ear. *You are never good enough, you won't be able to achieve that, why did you say that? You are so stupid...*

I say this with all the love in the world: those stories have been created by the 6-year-old version of you. Whilst she has done a beautiful job of keeping you safe, it is time for you to show her the way now. The truth is, she is safe to be the authentic expression of herself, to take risks, to set up a business, to do and honour all she desires because your soul *knows* you are capable of so much more. Your destiny is so much bigger than the safe life (prison) you have been keeping yourself in.

The ego is love. But love in a fucked up, upside down kind of way. It keeps you safe by creating stories which you buy into.

Believe me, the subconscious is really, really good at its job. It was designed for your survival, so it is masterful. It is dark, sneaky, and creeps up on you when you are not looking. I often think of my ego like Gollum, latching on to the doorway and pulling me back into the cave when I am taking a step forward. *Come here, my precious...*

Every time we dishonour and let ourselves down by staying stuck, the ego chimes in: "See – I told you." We consistently seek evidence to keep ourselves stuck and when we find that evidence (which we create ourselves by sabotaging things) we have all the more reason to not take action. It is the perfect practice of self-preservation but one thing is for sure, it does not make you happy. And what do you do when you are not happy? You seek comfort in things which are easier to find, like food. (And believe me, it is highly unlikely that comfort you seek will come in the form of a salad!)

We hold weight for all sorts of reasons, but always to keep us safe in some way. It is always coming from a place of upside down love.

Perhaps we are using food to seek comfort from the things we are avoiding, rather than taking action. Your job is to figure out what you need to feel safe and then to give yourself that safety.

Your ego holds patterns of self-preservation and your authentic self knows the truth of what you could really achieve, but my guess is you are not slowing down enough to listen to her right now.

Your authentic self is your truth. She is a goddess, queen, rock star, powerhouse. A loving nurturer in the full expression of her femininity, she is loving, compassionate, strong, capable, able, boundaried. She is your wisdom, your kindness, your love, your light. She wants you to be healthy as much as you want it.

Affirmations

- It is safe for me to take loving steps towards my goals
- It is safe for me to trust I am supported
- Things work out as I envision them
- I expect things to go better than I could possibly imagine

Exercise

Notice how your ego tells you stories that are unkind and untruthful. Become deeply aware of your internal dialogue. How often are you unkind to yourself? Start to notice and challenge the thoughts you have with love, and recognise these thoughts are coming from your younger self. It is very important to practice awareness with love. There is a little girl within you who is trying to keep you safe; be kind to her.

Practice observing the patterns you created to keep you safe when you were a little girl. Are the things you say to yourself really true? Ask yourself: is this a fact or actually, is it fiction? Where is the evidence for the things you have been telling yourself and is it time to talk to yourself differently?

Whenever I notice my ego come up and I feel fear, I take myself off somewhere quiet, put my hand on my heart and say "It's OK sweetheart, you are safe and you are doing great. Thank you for looking after me but I have got this. I will show you a different way, a gentle and loving way – we can do it together."

See if this lands for you and if it does, use it as often as you possibly can.

Uncaging Your Thoughts and Beliefs

"Your beliefs become your thoughts,
Your thoughts become your words,
Your words become your actions,
Your actions become your habits,
Your habits become your values,
Your values become your destiny."
- Gandhi

When the intention behind your actions comes from a place of self-love and nourishment, then true health will naturally follow. Ridding yourself of limiting beliefs is where healing truly begins.

We all hold both limiting and empowering beliefs. Our beliefs sit like a GPS system deep within our subconscious. We translate what we see, hear, and experience through our very own internal navigation system. We distort, delete, and generalise things so that they fit into what we already believe. If you have ever heard something completely different than someone else, even though you were listening to the same thing, that is a prime example.

Think of your mind like an iceberg. There's the 10% you are aware of. This is your logical brain; the part of your brain that decides, 'Today I will be good. I'm firmly on that wagon, I'll do this thing.' However, the bit we have forgotten to take into account is the subconscious mind. This makes up the other 90% of our mind – the bit that's under the water. It's invisible to the naked eye but actually has tremendous influence over that conscious 10%.

Your subconscious is made up of the beliefs you hold, which have been created though your childhood, informed by society, or passed down through ancestral lines. The times when your Mum might have been too busy to spend time with you, the way your Dad spoke to you, how your teacher humiliated you in class one day – you made meaning out of all of those experiences. Meanings like *I am not loveable, I am not good enough, I am not worthy.* Whilst the meaning you made is not true, you have carried those beliefs your whole life and created your whole life experience from those beliefs.

Subconscious programmes run 95-99% of our daily behaviour and habits. Many of the programmes you run were created before you even turned 6. The meaning you made of those early experiences, however, does not have to shape your choices and experiences today. You can find those beliefs and change them. What a travesty if you live your whole life from untrue meanings you created when you were a child, which prevent you from shining and sharing your brightness with the world.

In order to create change in your life, you have to get that 90% of your mind on board with where you want to go. The beliefs you hold, which your mind believes are keeping you safe, ultimately keep you stuck in a false idea of comfort – which in reality is not comfortable at all but miserable.

My coach Gina, who loves a good metaphor, likened change to a hermit crab and I loved that image so much I am going to share it with you. When a hermit crab outgrows its shell, it has to make the brave decision to leave that shell and find another one, otherwise it will go through great pain and ultimately die. Leaving the shell takes courage. It has to venture out without any protection, utterly vulnerable, to find a new shell. The choice it faces: stay and die or find courage to go out and find a new and bigger home for its expansion. Of course, once it finds its new home, there is safety once again. It's only the bit in between that feels unknown and risky.

The same goes for you. You will find new safety when you make change, but first you have to find courage.

What are you ready to let go? What have you been telling yourself for years which is simply not true?

A really common belief is 'I am not good enough' or 'I am not worthy' which of course you now know is not true. Other common beliefs include 'If I achieve what I desire, I will not be loveable', 'Being the weight I want to be makes others uncomfortable', 'I am loveable when I am unhealthy because then I get attention'.

There are all sorts of beliefs which sit in the depths of our mind. They might not make sense to the logical mind and the part of you that simply wants to move forward – but in order to heal it is essential you find them and teach yourself it is safe to let them go.

I often think of humans as walking around with a cage around their heads - caged by their own thoughts and beliefs. If they simply took those cages off, they would see the world in a completely different way.

Please remember, however, that your cage was put there to keep you safe. It is important to remove it with great care. Being cruel or hard on yourself will only tighten the cage. Healing, learning, and growth is a process and it must be done with care, gentleness, and love.

One of my teachers once said to me, "You are not your thoughts," which blew my mind. I had never seen it that way before. I had never realised that was not who I was. I had never realised that I was in fact the observer of my thoughts, and if I had a head full of thoughts, well, I could actively pick ones that served me!

I have heard hundreds of women say, "I always thought I had horrible legs." This is a really common belief! I thought this about myself too – for years, it kept me stuck and meant I didn't wear shorts and hid in jeans on exceptionally hot days. How I suffered as I watched the women with "lovely" legs enjoy their cool shorts. I have since been shocked to hear how many other women have felt the same their whole lives. The saddest part is, many are in their 50s and 60s. Now they say, "When I look at old photos of myself, I realise there was absolutely nothing wrong with my legs at all." It was simply a belief that restricted them for their whole lives.

It is thoughts like these that no longer serve you well. The problem is that the thoughts you keep thinking become a belief - and when you believe something you will keep acting it out, making it your reality. It is time to dig them out and burn them to the ground, giving you the freedom to create a new image of yourself.

Select only thoughts to keep that stem from a place of truth, love, and authenticity. You have to take a surgeon's knife to your thoughts, carefully dissecting them. Remember, many of your patterns were created as a child to keep you safe. Now it's time for you to parent yourself with love and kindness and, from your adult self, let those old thoughts go.

From now on, you are the goddess warrior guardian of your subconscious. You are responsible for what you let into that brain of yours. Whatever you keep letting in, you will start to believe. It's totally possible to change beliefs later, but honestly, it is way easier to vet those thoughts in the first place.

Test your thoughts and beliefs. Ask yourself: Is this fact or fiction? What evidence do I have to tell me this is real? What evidence do I have to negate this story I am telling myself?

Affirmations

- All my beliefs are in alignment with my goals

- Because of my empowering beliefs, I know that anything is possible

- By constantly repeating my desires, I create perfect belief in my ability to reach them

- Every day I edit and improve my beliefs

- I examine my past beliefs and release those which no longer serve me.

- I replace past limiting beliefs with new empowering ones

- I accept that my current circumstances are mirrors that indicate my current belief system

Exercise 1
Explore the beliefs that are no longer serving you

Sit down with your journal and spend some time thinking about what beliefs you carry and which ones hold you back. When we strip it right back, we tend to have one core limiting belief that we then create lots of sub-beliefs from. Once you find your core limiting belief, you will be able to identify how it shows up on a daily basis. It will influence your relationships, behaviour, career, how you parent, your finances, everything in your life.

It can take time to uncover all your beliefs and sometimes it might be a good idea to get help from a coach. That said, it might be very obvious to you when you begin to think about it. Start to ask yourself questions about where the same pattern keeps playing out in your life and why.

Take a look at these examples of core limiting beliefs. Several may resonate, but is there one core belief you can identify?

- I am unworthy
- I am unloveable
- The world is not a safe place
- People are not trustworthy
- I am undeserving
- I am incapable
- I am misunderstood
- I am always abandoned
- I am a victim
- I am a burden
- I am not clever
- I am bad
- I am always guilty

- I am powerless

- I am unattractive

- I am separated from God

- I am sinful

- I am a failure

Once you have identified your core belief and sub-beliefs, journal about where it has held you back in your life and what you are ready to believe instead. These limiting beliefs are not true. They are simply the result of a meaning you made out of a childhood experience, and they have been influencing your life for far too long. It is time to let them go and rewrite your story.

What do you want life to look like instead? Write out your new beliefs in your journal and reflect on what new patterns you would like to create.

Exercise 2
Letter to the little girl version of you

The second exercise in this section is to write a letter to your younger self. This is a very powerful exercise, so if you have experienced trauma that has not been processed, I recommend you seek out a good therapist or trauma specialist before doing this.

When you feel ready, write a letter to the little girl version of you. Maybe she is 6, maybe she is younger or older – you will feel called to the age that is right for you. Take time to tell her about all the things you would like her to know that she didn't realise then: her innocence, her capability, how special she is, how pure her heart is. Tell her everything a little girl should know about herself. Share with her your wisdom from this future version of yourself. Take your time with this exercise; it is very important not to rush it. Imagine you are sitting with her and you have the opportunity to tell her everything that you would if you were parenting her.

When you think of yourself as that innocent and wonderful little girl, how could you ever think you are not enough? How could you ever be horrible to yourself? She is you. She needs your love.

Your Inner Dialogue

The way you speak to yourself matters more than you could ever know. In fact, it could be argued that it is the most important thing you could ever do. If you are negative, critical, and consistently giving yourself a hard time, the way you communicate will settle into your subconscious and become your reality. Everything we are working towards in this book is about creating joy in your life, and that has to start from within.

Happiness is not found outside of yourself; it is created by you. You create your own reality through what you think. If you focus on the negative, if you constantly worry about what might go wrong or fear what people think of you, guess what? Besides being a very stressful way of living, this will only amplify your worries and fears. Think about it for a moment. How are worry, criticism, negativity, and judgement ever going to help you achieve the things you desire? Negativity feeds itself and only creates more negativity as a result.

It is not possible to experience joy if you are busy focusing on all that is wrong all of the time. What I'm about to say might make you cringe, but you need to have a love affair with yourself. You need to fall madly in love with who you are, celebrate who you are, and imagine you are talking to that very special little girl whom you just found through your letter writing in the last exercise. Any words you now speak need to come from her.

My internal dialogue used to be appalling. *I am fat, I am ugly, I am not good enough, I am unhappy, I am lonely, I have disgusting skin…*

Simply writing them out now makes me feel miserable.

Take a moment to think about your internal dialogue. Is it similar to mine? What do you think about your body? How do you talk to it?

I expect your thoughts go something along the lines of *I feel heavy, I am fat, I need to lose weight, I am unattractive.* Just say those words out loud for a moment. Think about how often you think them. How do those words make you feel?

Every day I receive hundreds of emails from women with statements like these below. I have not edited any of them; they are written exactly as I have received them and only make up a very small selection of what I consistently read:

- I have let myself down by not staying fit & healthy after losing weight & putting it back on again.

What's the point in exercising and slimming again - no one sees me anyway?

- My flabby stomach shows way too much in my clothes

- I am disgusting

- I can't be bothered

- I will always overeat

- I don't like the view in the mirror

- I always quit after about two months of being determined

- I hate my body

- I hate myself and what I see in the mirror

- I hate my love for bad things

- I hate what I look like in photos

- I am lumpy and chunky

- I don't feel sexy

- I never stick to good eating habits

- I eat and drink things with little or no nutrition

- I'm lazy

- I have no motivation

- I feel sorry for myself

- I obsess over food and eating

- I wear baggy frumpy clothes and I would like to have more body confidence to wear more fashionable clothes.

- I have no faith in my own abilities

They are heart-breaking to read, aren't they? It is devastating to me that a huge proportion of women are living with these thoughts every day as I used to as well.. If you relate to this kind of language and self-talk, know that you are not alone, and it is absolutely possible for you to transform your life. I know, because I did and that means you can too.

You might be thinking that you can't possibly believe anything positive about yourself. I hear you. We are going to take baby steps and create statements that you can work with right now. From there, you can let them grow. You might not feel aligned with saying, "I am the perfect weight for my body" right now. Find the next best thought that feels good when you think it, something like:

- It feels good for me to take care of my body

- My body loves to be nourished

- I am taking steps towards loving my body a little more every day

- My body gives me life and in return, I take care of it

- My body knows how to be healthy

The words you put after I or I AM are essential to your wellbeing. They become your identity. Your mind believes what you tell it. You HAVE to understand this!

I bet you have got some clearing up to do around your language and beliefs in relation to the miraculous machine you live in. The truth is – you are incredible. You are not any of the things you have been telling yourself. That is not WHO you are. It's time to dive deep into the beliefs and language you have been using and start shifting toward a loving, kind, and accepting way of speaking to yourself.

Transformation of any kind starts the other way around from the way I expect you have been approaching it. If you want to create anything in your life, you have to stop thinking negatively about it, and that you will only be happy when you have it.

Your positive thought has to come first. That positive thought creates the vibration through which you create your reality.

However, you need to do more than just think your new thoughts in your head – you need to *feel* them. If you don't feel good right now, how is that going to help you get to where you want to be? Stop basing your happiness on an external situation and instead allow yourself to feel good in the moment and create life from there. It really doesn't matter what your current reality is. If you want to make change in your life, you are going to have to change the way you think and how you speak to yourself. You have been led to believe you are happy when you achieve something, the reality is, creation comes from you being happy first.

You need to get into the energy of feeling good and no-ticing joy in each moment is the most powerful tool you have. It will change your life.

I am not enormously fond of the word gratitude. If you are not careful, gratitude can be used to compare: 'at least my life is not as bad as theirs', 'at least my life is better than it was then', 'at least I don't look too bad'. This is not gratitude. It is actually judgement, and it is taking you right back into the low vibration you are working to get out of.

Instead I really like the word appreciation because it has a slightly different energy. Take a moment, breathe deep, and reflect. What do you appreciate in your life now? What you are sitting on? That you have eyes to read these words? That you have hands to hold this book? That you are alive? What can you hear? Can you hear the birds sing-ing? Can you hear silence? What does that sound like? Appreciation is found in slowing down and moving into the present.

I once heard a story about Warren Buffet going into a room of adolescents and telling them: "I am going to give you all a car. Whatever car you want, you can have it – it's yours, but it comes with some conditions. It will be the only car you ever have. You can't sell it or replace it. It will be yours for the rest of your life.

"How will you look after it?"

They all replied with how well they would service it, cherish it, wash it, polish it, etc.

And then he said, "OK, I am not going to give you each a car, but you have that already in your body and mind. They are the most precious things you will ever own. Look after them because they are what you experience your life through and the quality of your life is determined by how well you look after them."

Wow – I love that! It shifts your perspective, doesn't it?

Your body is the engine through which you experience life. It is so very keen for you to love it and the more you do, the more it will be what you want it to be.

What DO you appreciate about your body? If you didn't have it, you wouldn't here, so it is a pretty special gift you are sitting in right there.

Did you know it is impossible to feel in a low vibration mood and be in an energy of appreciation at the same time? It's true!

If you stay in the energy of appreciation more often than the energy of lack, I promise your life will change in ways beyond your wildest dreams. If you don't believe me right now, just try it – what have you got to lose?

Affirmations

- I take time every day to get into the energy of appreciation

- I appreciate with wonder the life I am surrounded by

- I notice the joy around me every day

- I am deeply grateful for the life I experience through the amazing body I live in

Exercise

Practice appreciation as part of your daily routine. Start every morning by focusing deeply on what you are grateful for or appreciative of. It doesn't have to take up a huge amount of your time. To create change in your life, you absolutely have to change the way you think. If you start every day by waking up and thinking the same thoughts as yesterday, then you are going to struggle to change your life. First thing in the morning is the best time to practice appreciation (even better if you practice all day!). As soon as you wake up in the morning – direct your thoughts to appreciation and everything you are grateful for – notice the shift in your energy. Try thoughts like:

- 'I appreciate my warm and comfortable bed'

- 'I appreciate I have warm water in my bathroom'

- 'I appreciate the feeling of water touching my skin in the shower'

- 'I appreciate my feet touching the ground as I get up and taking me through the day'

- 'I appreciate the laundry I have to do, it means I have clothes to wear'

- 'I appreciate the dishes, it means I have food and mouths to feed'

To start, I suggest choosing three things – one big and two small – to focus on, so that you get used to becoming appreciative of everything around you all of the time.

Enjoy this process. It is a beautiful one that I could write a whole book about. Perhaps that will be the subject of my next book!

Welcoming and Experiencing All Emotions

Your external world will not change until you change the way you see it from your internal world. Everything is about perspective. The way you experience your world is a choice. You hold the most beautiful magic key to your happiness. It sits within you. Your happiness and joy is not dependent on what happens outside of you; that belief gives all of your power away. You have so much more power than you can possibly imagine.

We are not taught about emotions at school, even though these are the very things that drive our life experience. The reason you eat, the reason you make any choice, the reason you do all that you do is because of how you feel. It is not logic that determines these things, but emotion.

Humans are meaning making machines. We make meaning of all of our experiences and interactions. Something happens in our external world and we see it through our own individual lens and belief system. We interpret something someone said to us or something that happened based on our own perspective of the world. Effectively, we validate our limiting beliefs through interpretation and that creates feelings such as sadness, grief, and jealousy.

For example, if you believe that you are not good enough, your mind will be looking to reinforce this belief and will seek all the evidence it can find to prove it true. Once you have the evidence, the emotion will follow. Not feeling good enough is of course going to result in low vibration feelings such as sadness, grief, jealousy and anger. They sprout up like weeds in the garden and if you don't keep your mind weed-free, those emotions will become your normal.

If we don't know that this is happening, and we don't know that we can guide ourselves toward happier emotions, we will let those negative feelings control and confine us. We will live a life not of choice and free will but one determined by the habits of our mind and the emotions it causes us to feel.

In fact, life does not happen to you. You make it happen *for* you.

You can learn to direct how you feel. You have the power to do that and create freedom and joy. Your mind becomes a servant to you rather than something which is controlling you.

The process is not about ignoring your emotions or pushing them down. After all, to be human is to experience a range of emotions. Instead it is about listening to them and honouring them. As children we are taught that low vibration emotions are not welcome – anger, sadness, jealousy, worry. Our parents don't want us to feel these things; they want their children to be happy! As children we are often guided out of truly sitting with our feelings (sometimes with the bribe of food!) so we learn to push them down and ignore them because we are taught they are not acceptable. We learn to hide them behind a smile. How many times have you said "I'm fine" when you are breaking apart inside?

I often think of emotions like skin. Your skin is full of nerves to stop you hurting yourself; if you didn't feel, you wouldn't know if you were burning yourself. Your emotions are the same. They are your guide.

The truth is, no emotion is bad. They are all welcome. They are all telling you something. No matter why you are experiencing them or the belief which has driven them, they are your current experience and that is extremely valid. However, you are not stuck with them. You can use them as a guide to understand more deeply what you need.

I think of it like inviting the negative parts of myself to my dinner table, where irritation, frustration, anger, fear are all welcome. I take time to get to know them like old friends, asking questions and searching more deeply without judging or criticising. I ask them why they're here, where they came from, and what they need.

Low vibration emotions usually come from a younger part of ourselves needing to be heard; perhaps a 6-year-old feeling unloved, or a defiant teenager feeling misunderstood. Our subconscious holds all these parts of ourselves and keeps playing out the same patterns until we learn to welcome and love them.

Healing is always found in love. Next time you feel low, welcome those feelings with open arms and ask what they need – just like you would offer kindness to a little girl. Offer yourself love and see what your feelings have to say in return. They need love, attention, and understanding. Sit with them instead of pushing them down or numbing them.

Have you ever been told to "be more positive" when you are sad? It is triggering isn't it! If you dishonour or ignore your emotions you will keep experiencing them. It is important to validate what you feel, understand where it is coming from and as you do so, you can move through it. Hard emotions are not about anything you have done wrong. Allowing yourself to feel them and be with them is the key to healing.

The Abraham-Hicks Levels of Emotion scale lists the 22 most commonly felt emotions in order of how good they feel. Low vibration feelings are at the bottom and high vibration feelings are at the top.

1. Joy/Appreciation/Empowered/Freedom/Love
2. Passion

3. Enthusiasm/Eagerness/Happiness

4. Positive Expectation/Belief

5. Optimism

6. Hopefulness

7. Contentment

8. Boredom

9. Pessimism

10. Frustration/Irritation/Impatience

11. Overwhelment

12. Disappointment

13. Doubt

14. Worry

15. Blame

16. Discouragement

17. Anger

18. Revenge

19. Hatred/Rage

20. Jealousy

21. Insecurity/Guilt/Unworthiness

22. Fear/Grief/Depression/Despair/Powerlessness

It's a powerful tool to use in understanding and moving through your emotions.

Let's say you feel guilt (emotion #21). You wouldn't expect to jump up to #1 at once. It would be very hard to do that, and would put too much expectation on you – probably pushing you down the levels even further.

Instead, you could think about what thoughts and beliefs created guilt within you. Once you have explored the emotion, you can work toward moving up a level or two by identifying your next best thought. It is necessary to move through the levels of emotion to get you back up to high vibration feelings. For example, when you get to anger (#17), you can the work on identifying feelings of worry (#14) and working through those. Every emotion is an improvement on the one you felt before and you will always naturally want to work up towards #1: Joy/Appreciation/Empowered/Freedom/Love.

Instead of trying to just get over it and be happy, you are naming your emotions, owning them, accepting them, and then letting them go, one emotion at a time until you feel better.

Don't let yourself stay on the lower part of the emotional scale for too long. You can make yourself feel differently with the right kind of thoughts. Remember, naturally your state is joyful and loving. When you feel good, you are in higher alignment with yourself and when you feel low, you are out of alignment with the truth of who you are – that is why it doesn't feel good. Instead of allowing lower vibration feelings to become your identity, ask what they are teaching or showing you. If you are feeling anxious, what is the emotion behind it? Is there fear of not being loved or accepted hiding in there?

Behind every behaviour there is an emotion. There is always a reason behind why you do what you do; your job is to figure out why so that you can change your behaviour.

For example, as I write these words for you, I cycle through phases of feeling stuck, struggling to explain what I mean in ways that would be helpful and easy to understand. My mind then creates stories (*see, you shouldn't even try to write a book, you will never get it done!*) and then my emotion follows – feeling insecure and unworthy. Before I was aware of any of this, the next step for the old me would have been to numb those feelings with food because they don't feel good.

Instead, I slow down and ask myself what I am feeling. I ask myself what would get me into a higher vibration and what my next best thought could be. I tell myself writing is a process and what I really need is a break, a change of scenery, so I can come back to writing with a fresh perspective.

Rather than letting your emotions determine your experience, use your emotions to guide you toward a better thought. Choose thoughts that allow you to rise up the scale.

Affirmations

- I am allowed to feel this way

- I am not defined by what I feel

- I use my emotions as a signpost to direct me towards my needs and desires

- This experience doesn't control me

- This feeling doesn't have to determine my whole day.

- The greatest gift I can give myself is the awareness of what I need right now

- The inner work that I do directly benefits the people around me as well as myself

- Even though I feel like this, I am OK

- Even though I feel like this, I am worthy of love and respect

- I wonder what this feeling wants me to see

Exercise

Practice recognising and honouring your emotions rather than pushing them down or ignoring them. Understand that they are guiding you toward your needs. Try using the levels of emotion scale to guide you through what you feel. Notice as you go up and down the levels and ask yourself what the next best feeling or thought would be? Even if you are moving from guilt to anger – recognise that as a healing step, moving you closer to joyful emotion.

Other great questions to ask are:

- How could this be working out *for* me?
- What do I really need right now?

You Have Permission

For most of my life, I was waiting for someone to tell me I was good enough. Waiting to be saved and given permission to be who I was. I lived in the world of 'when I...' *When I am this thin, when I look like that, when I weigh this much, when I have a boyfriend, when my son is older, when I have more money - when, when, when, when.*

I realise now they were all stories I had created as ways to keep myself nice and safe in my comfort zone but the thing is, the comfort zone isn't very comfortable, is it? It is actually pretty miserable.

My message to you is stop waiting for someone to tell you what you are looking for, because they are not coming. The person you are looking for is you. You have permission to shine. The permission comes from within. What are you waiting for?

No one is going to come and tell you it is time, no one is going to come and save you, no one is going to come and say you are ready and in actual fact, you are probably never going to be ready – you just have to take that leap of faith and go for it.

A couple of years ago, I woke up at 3am and felt a calling to get on my meditation mat. I really didn't want to get out of bed, as it was a cold and dark winter morning, yet I had this really strong urge to meditate. So, despite every part of me wanting to go back to sleep, I did as I was 'being told'!

I got up, went and sat in my meditation space, and as I moved into meditation, I clearly heard the words: "Let go of the fear of judgement so that you can hear me and do my work."

Those words have stayed with me ever since and I have been working on them hard, with coaches, meditation, prayer. It has not been easy. There have been a lot of tears, a lot of heaviness and darkness. I even spent a day with a Shaman to help me clear ancestral and childhood trauma.

But what I realised through this work is I have kept myself safe, stuck and small for fear of judgement. *What will others think? Who am I to have an opinion on this? Who am I to be successful and have everything?*

This brings us right back to that Marianne Williamson quote: "Who are you not to be?"

You simply have permission to be awesome because you are. The chances of you even being born were one in four trillion. That is scientific proof that you are, quite literally, a miracle. So, you have permission to live your life like you are a goddamn miracle – because you are. You are inherently amazing. It is as simple as that!

I know that is true because we all are. My belief is that everyone is incredible, and everyone is full of potential and love.

(Sometimes people get disconnected from that truth. Through their childhood conditioning they might have created beliefs that they are not good enough or lovable and that can mean they BEHAVE in a way which is not in alignment to the truth of who they are. Certainly – people's behaviour can be despicable, unkind, and unloving, but that is not their identity. It means they are lost and unhappy and from that place they may do unkind things.)

The more you move into alignment with yourself and truly love and accept who you are, the more you can take action from this place of truth. It is not your job to compare yourself to anyone else. Where you are right now is perfect. Take steps which serve you from where you are. You know the difference when you are taking action from a place of alignment because it feels good and you feel excited – judgement and comparison simply fall away.

The reality is, you have permission to live your very best life. You have permission to shine. You have permission to be successful (in whatever way that means to you). You have permission to be happy. You have permission to be healthy. You have permission to RISE UP.

In fact, you have permission to…

- Change your career
- Laugh just because
- Dance like no one is watching
- Go out for dinner alone
- Take a day off
- Potter
- Do nothing
- Not do the laundry
- Call an old friend
- Dump an old friend
- Cry
- Use your best crockery
- Wear a dress for no reason
- Go out without makeup
- Go out with makeup
- Swim naked
- Learn a new language
- Take a day off and watch old films
- Get a cleaner
- Ask your partner to cook their own dinner
- Follow your heart

- Book a holiday on your own

- Learn an instrument

- Sing loudly

- Wear colour

- Say no

- Say yes

- Shout in the woods

- Receive pleasure

- Love sex

- Be sexual

- Be in your empowered feminine

- Be vulnerable

- Ask for help

- Not know the answer

- Know the answer

- Use your intuition

- Not know facts but trust your feelings

- Cry

- Say what you are thinking

- Tell someone you love them

Stop looking over at someone else's lane and focus on your own. It really doesn't matter what other people think. What do YOU think?

Clara, a wonderful lady I once worked with, spoke of seeking permission outside of herself. She said, "I have lived in so much doubt and fear. I always questioned everything. Should I? Shouldn't I? What will others think? Will others approve? I needed permission from everything and everybody outside of myself and in actual fact, the only person who needed to show up for me, was me. I needed to give myself permission to live freely in my own right as an expression of the individual that I am."

Those feelings you are searching for aren't going to come from somewhere new, someone special, or something wonderful. They're going to come from deep within you, where they are patiently waiting for you to give yourself permission to be released. Joy, happiness, and freedom are not things that happen to you. They happen because they are who you are – your job is to simply tap in and allow yourself to feel and express them.

One of the most life-changing books I have ever read is Man's Search For Meaning by Victor Frankl. A quote from that book that has left a profound impact on me is:

"When we are no longer able to change a situation, we are challenged to change ourselves.

Everything can be taken from a man but one thing: the last of the human freedoms—to choose one's attitude in any given set of circumstances, to choose one's own way. Between stimulus and response there is a space. In that space is our power to choose our response. In our response lies our growth and our freedom."

Victor Frankl was a prisoner in Auschwitz, where he lost his father, mother, brother, and wife. If someone who goes through something like that can recognize that despite everything he lost and everything he experienced, he still had the ability to choose his attitude, he didn't need to wait for permission from anyone, and he was not defined by that experience but used it to find his inner strength and capability…then we can do that too.

Stop waiting for conditions to be perfect. Stop waiting to be saved. Stop waiting until you are thin enough. Stop waiting. It will never come. Now is the time. You have permission.

You have permission to be a woman. To be in your sexual power. To own your femininity. To receive pleasure. To love yourself. To nourish yourself.

You cannot become what you are not willing to be vibrationally right now. The more you allow yourself to be who you truly are, the more of what you seek will come to you. It doesn't come through waiting until, it comes through being now.

Affirmations

- I have permission to express myself from a place of authenticity

- I have permission to be myself

- I give myself permission to create more balance, bliss, and brilliance in my life

- I give myself permission to shine

Exercise

Write a letter from your future 100-year-old self to you now.

When your future self is looking back over her life from a place of wisdom, what does she want this version of you to know? What does she want to say to you?

Describe what life has been like, and how grateful she is to you for taking the steps you did to enable her to have the life she has had. How amazing has her life been? What did she go on to achieve? What did you experience? What messages of wisdom does she have to share with you?

This is a really beautiful and powerful exercise. Take your time with it. Write it from a place of nurturing love. Take yourself forward to that future version of yourself, when you are looking back over your life, and speak from her to you now.

Good Girl, Bad Girl

How often have you said or heard your friends say "I am trying to be good at the moment"? I would put my money on literally thousands.

As women we are deeply conditioned to be 'good girls'.

"Be a good girl and..."

Did your mother say that to you? Maybe your teacher? Or maybe you have even heard yourself say it to your daughter?

We have also been conditioned to believe that it is socially acceptable to only look a certain way. Images of this ideal have been lasered into the back of our minds from a dangerously young and impressionable age. Dolls, magazines, princesses, film stars, TV...even well known cartoon characters in their little outfits! An endless stream telling us that this is what we should look like' leaving many women with a chronic dose of 'comparisonitis'.

Whilst you may not consciously be aware of your conditioning, it is running a continuous loop in your subconscious - like a cassette going around and around and around. Humans have approximately 90,000 thoughts a day and about 95% of those thoughts are the same. Every single day. That's an awful lot of days played out with the same unconscious conditioning barrage... and there we are blaming our willpower!

Combine this fundamental need to be a 'good girl' with the incessant social conditioning and our own habit loop mindsets, and we become deeply programmed. At a sub-conscious level we believe that our worth is measured by things outside of ourselves. In my opinion, this is one of the most damaging beliefs society instils in us.

You are simply wonderfully worthy. You just are. You came into this world truly beautiful and full of potential; nothing about that fact has changed. Sometimes we lose a sense of our true identity in the hustle and bustle of life. Our minds become so full of what everyone else thinks we should think that we lose connection from the inner knowing of our hearts.

You were born with the most insane amount of inherent worth and feminine wisdom. If you can recognise this and understand that it is yours for the taking when you tune into it, your life will change beyond belief.

The battles that are keeping you stuck in patterns that are no longer serving you will simply slip away. You don't have to try to beat the cycle. Instead, focus on letting go and simply remembering who you are.

It's time to lose the 'good' and 'bad' food day labels immediately. No longer are you going to give your power away to these statements.

Your day is not defined by what you ate.

Labelling a day as a 'good' or 'bad' food day is dangerously close to labelling yourself as 'good' or 'bad'. To diminish yourself to being good or bad because of the food you ate is doing yourself a serious disservice.

Nothing you put in your mouth ever makes you a bad person. Equally – having a 'good' food day does not make you holier than thou. So the healthy eating police can get off their high horses too!

Your self-worth has nothing, and I mean NOTHING, to do with the number on the scales or what you choose to eat. Your self-worth comes from a much deeper place.

You will have come to realise by now this is not your typical weight loss book. It doesn't contain a food plan. Instead, it gives you permission to be the goddess that you are. That is where true health and wellness are found…in treating yourself as you deserve to be treated.

Before we go any further, let's address the 'wagon'. Remember, this is a myth! You are never 'on' or 'off' a health wagon.

Health is about building a loving relationship with our bodies. We need to learn how to nurture our body, mind, and soul with the food we eat, the thoughts we have, and the actions we take.

Of course, our bodies need nutrients to be able to carry out the cellular processing we need to thrive. Thyroid function, weight, clarity of thought, happiness levels, immunity, fertility, hormonal balancing and much more are all dependent on receiving nutrients that allow these processes to happen.

That said, you can eat all the nutrients in the world, but if you feel restricted by your diet it won't be long before you find yourself unhappy. As a result, you will lean towards making choices that don't feel good emotionally or physically.

The trick is finding balance with compassion towards yourself. This isn't a quick fix; your relationship with health and weight is a lifelong one.

So let's give the wagon a shove off the cliff. There is no wagon and there are no 'good' or 'bad' food days. Those concepts are over. We have a new focus now.

Your soul needs nourishment. Mostly that comes through foods that give you energy and help you feel full of health and vitality. Sometimes that will be a big old slice of chocolate cake, served without the sides of guilt, shame or judgement.

Affirmations

- I love and accept myself
- I am a special person. There's nobody else like me
- I love myself more and more each day
- I am worthy of love
- I am worthy of happiness

Exercise

We are going to start to uncover some of the long-held beliefs and stories you have been carrying around with you for years – it is time to take them out of the heavy backpack you carry around with you and lighten the load. Take some time to journal answers to the following questions to become aware of the beliefs you carry and how they drive your actions:

- What were you taught about food as a child?
- What was your relationship with food as a child?
- Was there plenty of food?
- What messaging did you receive around your body as a child?
- What was your Mum's relationship with food and her body like?
- How did your Mum talk about her body in front of you?
- How did your family talk about your body to you?

- What are your triggers when it comes to eating?

- Do you recognise any emotions that trigger you to eat?

- What has dieting taught you about food?

- How would you describe your relationship with your body?

The Amazing Home You Live In

You live inside a walking, talking miracle. Your body is doing millions of things on your behalf so that you stay alive every single day. One of the most important things you can do when you start to work towards health is make friends with the beautiful machine you live in. I know you don't think of it as beautiful, but this is where you are wrong, my love. Your body is beautiful. It is amazing.

It is crying out for you to be best friends with it. It is desperate for you to pay attention, and guess what? If you start paying attention and looking after it, it will serve you with more energy, motivation, clarity of thought, and your weight will settle in a place that feels good for you. It really is that simple.

If you have been stuck in years of dieting like I had been, know it is not your fault. The approach you have been taught is all upside down. You have been waiting to achieve a certain weight or appearance when what your body is seeking all along is your love. When you realise it has been showing up for you every day like your best friend, never expecting anything back, despite the things you have filled it with and the way you have talked to it; when you realise it is so worthy of your own love and you start to nourish it with your words and your food, it will give you the very thing you have been seeking.

The shift you desire is waiting for you.

The woman you are longing to be…how does she treat her body? Be her now and you will achieve what you want.

Your body is always telling you what it needs; it's a constant whispering. Maybe you've just been too busy to hear it. You need to slow down, listen, and learn to deeply love who you are. It's time to nurture that wonderful machine that you live in and start looking after it. It is your energy centre, and the choices that you make around what you put into your body will either empower or disempower you.

We're currently facing one of the scariest eras in our lifetime. Health and wellbeing statistics are spiralling, with illnesses such as heart disease, cancers, diabetes and obesity rapidly rising. Yet at the same time, women are dieting more than ever.

There seems to be a correlation between when we began dieting in the 1970s, and when our collective weight started to increase. Poor diets are associated with 11 million deaths worldwide, according to the Lancet Global Burden of Disease study. The WHO has reported that worldwide obesity has nearly tripled since 1975.

In 2016, more than 1.9 billion adults 18 years and older were overweight. Of these, over 650 million were obese. That makes 39% of adults aged 18 and over, overweight, and 13% of those were clinically obese.

There are 7.5 billion people on this planet. But you are more than just a statistic. Never before in the whole history of humanity and never again in the future will there ever, ever be another person like you! Don't ever forget that you were born with a healthy body. You were born with no limiting beliefs. Anything is possible, and it still is.

You started out with one cell, and now your body is made of 50 trillion cells. They came together from the division of one single cell. Every minute, 300 million of your cells die. That's just a small fraction of those 50 trillion cells, all squashed together to make you who you are.

Your brain can hold five times as much information as the Encyclopaedia Britannica. Your nerve impulses travel at 170 miles per hour. Your brain holds the same amount of power as a 10 watt light bulb. Don't let it keep getting stuck in the same thought patterns. It likes to be challenged. It likes to be taken out of its comfort zone.

Your heart creates enough pressure to squirt blood a distance of 30 feet, and pumps blood around your 60,000 miles of veins and capillaries. Your heart pumps six quarts of blood circulating three times every minute. In one day, your blood travels up to 12,000 miles.

Your skin is the ultimate touchscreen. Each square centimetre of your skin, which is the body's biggest organ, includes 1,300 nerve cells, 9,000 nerve endings, 36 heat centres, 75 pressure centres, 100 sweat glands, three million cells and three yards of blood vessels.

Your eyes alone are a study in genius. Your eyes can distinguish up to a million coloured surfaces and take in more information than the largest existing telescope. You blink once every four seconds. That's because your eyelashes act as windshield wipers, keeping the dust and the grime out.

Your liver is working super hard, keeping you alive by clearing out your body. It has over 400 functions, including detoxification, protein synthesis and the production of biochemicals necessary for digestion. However, if you lost two-thirds of your liver from surgery or trauma, it would grow back to its original size in four weeks. Wow. That's amazing!

Take a breath. You breathe 17,000 breaths every single day. Your breath is more nutrient-rich than food and water. Without the ability to breathe, you would die much quicker than if you didn't eat or didn't drink. Your lungs are filled with thousands of microscopic capillaries and have the equivalent surface area to a tennis court to oxygenate blood, making it easier for this to take place and get oxygen where it needs to go.

You have a disposable stomach lining. The acid in your stomach is as strong as battery acid. If it touched your skin, it would burn you. Your stomach gets a brand-new lining every four days. Strong digestive acids quickly dissolve the mucous-like cells lining the walls of your stomach, so your body replaces them routinely before they are compromised.

Your body is regenerating cells every single day. That means that you have a whole new set of taste buds every 10 days, that you have new nails every six months. You have a whole new set of bones every 10 years and an entirely new heart every 20 years. That is mind blowing! Every 20 years, your heart has grown so many new cells that it has regenerated completely.

Your body is constantly hard at work to protect you. You may not even be aware, but it is always working to ensure that you don't contract diseases like cancer. Cancers form when cells are altered in a way which reprograms their DNA. Thousands of cells suffer cancer-causing lesions every day. The body sends enzymes around to find these cells and it fixes them before they turn into tumours. All this is going on beneath the surface!

Wow. Look at the walking magnificent miracle that you are. You have the most amazing machine already. It's irreplaceable, it is priceless, and it will serve you for your entire life. It will be healthy on your behalf, as long as you give it the nutrients it needs. If you look after yourself, your body will look after you. This is a two-way relationship; you will get out as much as you put in.

I like to think about nurturing and nourishing over punishing our body. And dieting falls firmly in the punishment category.

Ditch the diets and start taking great care of yourself in mind, body, and soul; enabling your amazing body to keep doing what it's doing. The fact is that diets don't work. We've got to work with our body rather than against it. However, we tend to be in the mindset of punishing the body that we live in, giving it a hard time because it's not what we want, yet continuously feeding it rubbish. We're setting ourselves up for failure and disappointment.

Affirmations

- My body deserves love

- I am perfect, whole, and complete just the way I am.

- I feed my body healthy nourishing food and give it healthy nourishing exercise because it deserves to be taken care of.

- I love and respect the body I live in

- My body is the home through which I experience my life

- My body wants me to be healthy and well

Exercise

This exercise might bring up some feelings of discomfort, which is all the more reason why it is so important to do.

Your task is to spend time looking in the mirror every day and to be kind to yourself instead of critical.

Start with your face. Look at yourself in your eyes and ask yourself how you are today. Can you tell yourself you love yourself? If not, why not? If you can't, you need to start practising – seriously, it will transform your life. You can do this practice when you are brushing your teeth. Start building a relationship with yourself. Tell yourself "I love you" on a daily basis, as often as possible.

Every time you catch yourself being unkind to your body, replace the thought with one that celebrates your body instead. If you didn't have this miraculous machine you lived in, you wouldn't be here. It works tirelessly for you every day and I promise you, as you start to love the body you live in, you will feel so much more joyful.

Are You Living From Your Red Zone?

We've established just how miraculous the human body is. It's just so smart! It's absolutely irreplaceable. Despite how much we chuck at it, how little attention we pay, it just keeps showing up for us and we take it for granted, don't we?

This amazing machine that you live in is working for you all of the time. And you have your two nervous systems to thank for that.

You have both a parasympathetic nervous system and a sympathetic nervous system. The parasympathetic nervous system is where you reach homeostasis. It's where your body is calm and relaxed, and your immune system is humming along. The body is synthesising vitamins and nutrients, managing your metabolism correctly. Your sympathetic nervous system, on the other hand, is where you are responding to the world around you.

To keep things simple, I'm going to call the parasympathetic nervous system the green zone, and the sympathetic nervous system the red zone.

Most of the time, you're operating from the green zone. When you go into a stress response, the red zone takes over.

What do I mean by a stress response?

Your body is a really, really clever organism. We have evolved with a stress response that has kept us alive up till now. A hundred thousand years ago, you would have needed that survival system when faced with something like coming up close and personal with a tiger. Your first instinct would be to run away! Your stress response kicks into gear. You automatically start running, and you don't stop until you're safe.

What is physically happening in your body when you feel stressed? It goes into the red zone when you perceive a threat, and that shuts down your immune system, your fertility system, your hormone balancing system, your metabolism, the whole shebang. All of those systems draw a lot of energy. you don't need them, for the time being, while you're running away from a tiger. You just need to fire up and run; everything gets shut down so you can channel all your energy into running instead. Then you go back to homeostasis, back to your green zone, back to whatever you were doing before. You're calm again, and all is well. It's a beautiful system.

Unfortunately, in the modern world, we are in a stress response more often than not. We're switching in and out of the red zone throughout the day. We get up in the morning, we check our phone, we check our email, we check our Facebook, we check our Instagram. We think about the kids, the family, and all the stuff we need to do. We're dealing with debt, illness, work, chores, and sometimes other pressures like divorce or redundancy… it's never-ending.

Now, the brain doesn't distinguish between stresses. It hasn't adapted to modern society. We don't get upgrades every year when our contracts run out - we're working with an older model here. The brain doesn't know that you're not dealing with a tiger, that you're not running for your life. It just shuts down your systems because it detects that you're under stress.

Stress can be a major factor in weight gain. Let me explain why. When you're in the green zone, you're taking energy from your fat burning store. It takes longer, and that's okay, because you're not in a rush. But when you're in your red zone, you need to get energy from somewhere fast. Your body can't take energy from fat when it is stressed, because it's not burning the fuel quick enough to allow you to run away.

We have about 2,500 calories of glycogen storage compared to 150,000 calories of fat storage – that's a relatively limited amount of glycogen to draw from. Glycogen is your quick release energy store – it is the energy your body keeps in your reserve to give you energy when you need it. By about 4pm we've used up the majority of those calories.

One of the most common things that I see with the women I work with is that they get hungry, and they fall off their diet plan around the middle of the afternoon. They get really tired or they start snacking. Now, that is a key sign that you are under stress! Your body sends out a hormone called ghrelin, which says, "Please, can you eat something? It needs to be something sugary and fast-releasing so that you can give me the energy that I need." And that is likely to be something that isn't healthy for you.

Remember, your body thinks that you're under threat! Your brain isn't able to decipher whether or not you're going to be eaten by a tiger, or whether you're just overwhelmed by all of the different work and life pressures that you're currently under. It only knows that you are feeling stressed, so it will behave in the same way as it would if your life was in danger.

Most women's instinct is then to beat themselves up, because they believe that they haven't got willpower. They believe they can't stick to something; they tend to blame themselves for their lack of resolve.

That is not true. It's not about willpower. Your body's instinct for self-preservation is much, much more powerful than any diet you might be consciously trying to stick to.

If you are stressed then your pituitary gland sends warning messages through your endocrine system – it is certainly not a time to have a baby when you are facing the perceived threat of being eaten by a tiger. So you stop releasing progesterone, a hormone responsible for anti-anxiety, anti-depression, and a diuretic. With less progesterone, you become oestrogen dominant, which results in symptoms such as weight gain around your hips, thighs and mid-section, insomnia, feeling low, exhaustion, and low libido. (If you are going through menopause (moving into your wisdom years!) then you will be producing less progesterone from your ovaries anyway. The other place your body produces progesterone is your adrenal glands, but if they are busy making adrenaline, then they will not be making progesterone.)

Remember, your body is your best friend. It is your temple. It is there to keep you alive. It doesn't want you to die. It doesn't want you to be sick. It's going to work hard on your behalf and do all it can to keep you alive.

Just because you might not feel stressed doesn't mean you aren't. You could just be so used to functioning from a state of stress response that it feels normal.

The fact is, many of us are in our stress response a lot of the time. It's our new normal. That's why it's essential to make sure that we're spending as much time in our green zone as possible throughout the day. Being in a constant state of stress has a major and direct impact on health. It impacts our menopausal symptoms, our fertility, our immune system, and makes us more prone to illness, from the common cold through to nasty diseases.

The Centre for Disease Control found that 110 million people die every year as a direct result of stress. That is seven people every two seconds. Heart disease, high blood pressure, diabetes, depression, and anxiety are just some of the things that stress can cause. Chronic stress leaves an imprint on your body. It creates inflammation - and that is the foundation for every age-related disease, including Alzheimer's and dementia.

What can you do about it?

As simple as it sounds, you can begin working with your breath. It's free, and basic, and therefore often overlooked. Your breath directly moves you between the parasympathetic and sympathetic zones. The red zone is all about breathing in the chest, releasing cortisol and releasing adrenaline. However, when you breathe through your diaphragm and into your belly, you release oxytocin. The body calms down and you move into your green zone. It really is that straightforward. The body is so quick to adapt to the environment around you, but by bringing awareness to it, you can change your physical response.

Most of us don't breathe correctly. We breathe into our chest; we're not used to belly breathing. When a baby is born, they instinctively breathe and expand their belly. But as women, we've been taught to hold our tummies in.

It's important to trigger your diaphragm when you're breathing in order to move into the green zone. Don't underestimate the power of breathing properly - you can literally shift between the zones by doing this. Once you are there, your body is going to start to move into fat burning, doing the things that your body is naturally designed to do, and it will help you to reach a healthy weight.

Affirmations

- I am calm and at ease

- Tomorrow will bring new opportunities

- This will pass

- I am able to identify what is within my control in this situation

- I have the resources I need to move through this stressful situation

- My breathing is anchored from within my core and this breathing is relaxing to my body and mind

- I am calm

- I am relaxed

Exercise

Close your eyes. Start to get a sense of the crown of your head and all the way down to the centre of your pelvis. Follow that direct line down your spine and start to notice any tension that may be held in the shoulders, maybe any tension in the jaw. And then start to bring your awareness to your breath, breathing in through the nose and out through the mouth.

Take a deep breath in and follow that breath all the way down, filling the whole of your belly, filling the back of your body, the side of your body.

On exhalation, allow every part of your body to soften and relax a little bit more deeply as you let go.

Breathe in, completely filling your body all the way down to your belly for a count of four, then retain your breath for a count of four, and let it go for a count of four.

Doing this for a 10-minute period once a day, a few times an hour, or even just when you notice you're overwhelmed, will move you from your red zone to your green zone and re-establish homeostasis. Try doing this before you go to sleep and see what a difference it makes.

The Food You Eat

Whilst this is not a book about dieting or telling you what to eat, it is important to recognise that there are certain foods that serve you better than others. Self-care includes eating things that are good for you and nourish your cells (although, sometimes the biggest act of self-care is eating an ice-cream with full permission to enjoy it without guilt or shame!).

I look at healing from two perspectives. There is healing in the body through the food you eat and healing in your mind through the steps you take to come home and love who you are.

Eating to nourish your cells instead of eating to lose weight will absolutely transform your health and your life experience because when you feel good, life is infinitely better! Believe me, I used to have a hangover pretty much every day and feeling well is A LOT more joyful! I couldn't believe how great I felt when I started to change my diet. It was unlike anything I had ever experienced before and is largely why I do what I do, because I want everyone to experience how fantastic they can feel when they eat well.

"The vast majority of conventional nutritionists and doctors have it mostly wrong when it comes to weight loss. Let's face it: if their advice were good and doable, we would all be thin and healthy by now. But as a general rule, it's not. And the mainstream media messages often confuse things even more. It is based on many food lies. And the biggest lie of them all is this: all calories are created equal." - Dr Mark Hyman

I am not going to promote any specific way of eating because I really don't think you need yet another diet book, and I believe it is so important you do not feel restricted. However, everything changed for me when I learned to both love myself and eat properly. One of the most life changing books I have ever read is The China Study by Colin T Campbell. If you are interested in finding out more about food and how to truly nourish your body – then this should be your first stop.

There are some simple things you can start to do now. One of the most important is to eat WAY more fruit and vegetables and a lot less processed food, meat, and dairy. You will be shocked at how much better you feel by simply making these shifts. I am not saying to go hardcore vegan, but I am saying vegetables are good for you, and I would put my money on the fact you don't eat enough of them. Hundreds of women tell me that they eat healthily but when we take a close look at what they are eating, that is actually far from the truth. The problem is, you have probably not been taught to eat properly, but to eat and count calories instead. And these are two entirely different things.

We are no longer interested in calories. From now on, stop looking at how many calories something contains and start looking at what ingredients it contains. The rule of thumb is that if it has more than five, it probably isn't very good for you. If something has a long shelf-life, that is also a good giveaway that it is not good for you. Basically if something has been prepared in a factory, wrapped in plastic, and contains an ingredient that you don't typically find in a kitchen at home (like emulsifiers, stabilisers, preservatives, bulking agents, flavourings and colourings) you can go by the rule of thumb that it is not good for your body. It might say it is on the packet, but it is not.

Processed foods are also designed to be addictive so that you buy more of them. Your health is not of any concern to these companies. These foods are designed to be hyper-palatable, which means they hit the sweet spot of flavour that fires up your brain so it urges you to eat more. The right combination of salt, fat, and sugar is addictive because once upon a time, if you had stumbled across a food like this, it would have been a good idea to eat lots of it for your survival. This is no longer the case and there is plenty more available, but your brain does not know that.

Not only are these foods highly addictive, completely nutrient deficient, and full of sugar and fat, which means you pile the pounds on even if you stick within your calorie quota – they are also incredibly bad for your brain function, hormone balance, liver function, immune system, and overall health.

Vegetables are bursting with all the nutrients your body needs for you to be well. When I first started eating more vegetables I honestly thought life would become very boring indeed. My idea of vegetables was boiled broccoli and carrots. Wow – what a world I was about to discover. Not only did I very quickly start to feel amazing but the food was truly delicious!

Most women I talk to are terrified of eating fruit. Dieting companies have brainwashed us into thinking that something which grew on our earth is more dangerous to eat than something that came out of a packet. Let's put the fruit myth to bed – you can eat fruit! It is good for you. Fruit is full of phytonutrients, which you need thousands of to be well. The sugar in fruit is very different from processed sugar, and it absolutely does not behave in the same way in your body. When you eat whole fruit, the sugar is also bound to the fibre which means you have a green light to eat it!

If you have been told not to eat fruit, another school of thought you might have been told to believe is not to eat avocadoes or nuts. This is SO wrong! These are the best sources of fat. It is really important to reduce the amount of saturated fat you eat (a great way of recognising saturated fat is that it's solid at room temperature – so from animals) and eat more unprocessed plant-based fats. Omega 3s, which are essential for your brain health, can be found in these sources, as well as in flaxseeds and chia seeds – it's a great idea to add these to your smoothie or porridge in the morning.

Let's talk for a moment about carbohydrates. Carbs DON'T make you fat!

People often think that carbohydrates are not a healthy thing to consume. They have such a bad rep because there's so much misunderstanding of what they are. Really, it's just a matter of eating the right types.

There are simple carbohydrates, found in white bread, pasta, and chocolate. Then there are carbohydrates found in foods like whole grains, beans, legumes, pulses, and vegetables. These carbohydrates are also known as fibre and you need to eat plenty of them. This in itself will have a transformational impact on how you feel, your energy, and weight.

Fibre is essential to maintaining gut health. (Did you know that 80% of our serotonin, our happy hormones, comes from our gut? What better reason to look after it?) A whopping 90% of the UK's population is not eating enough fibre, which directly correlates to the huge increase in colon cancer.

When you eat a lot of processed foods, unhealthy bacteria weaken your gut wall. The lining of your digestive system is just one cell wide. When you eat poorly, it degrades those cells and they start to come apart. That means food can start to escape, which prompts your immune system to come and jump on that food, and that can lead to food intolerances.

This is why it is essential to eat lots of fruits and vegetables. The fibre intake from the complex carbohydrates they contain plays a crucial role in balancing our blood sugar and ensuring our gut health is optimal. If we don't get enough fibre in, then food sits and rots in our gut.

It's hard for our bodies to break down fibre. If you think about simple carbohydrates, there's no work for the body to do to extract the energy. For example, a chocolate bar has already started to break down in your mouth; your body didn't have to do anything to release those sugars. It just takes all that energy and stores it as fat. The body then releases insulin to try and mop the sugar up out of our bloodstream. This results in insulin resistance and ultimately diabetes, as a result of eating too many of the wrong kinds of carbohydrates.

When they said to eat a rainbow, they were right.

Let's take a look at some food myths and facts.

Myth: Restrictive Diets Work

I believe this is one of the most destructive lies we have been told. It is doing a great disservice to our bodies and our mental health and wellbeing. When we cut off nutrients we are cutting off vital nourishment to ourselves - all in the pursuit of feeling worthy. How does that even make sense? We torture ourselves through punishment and restriction, trying to achieve the desired outcome of finally feeling good enough. Malnutrition is not something that is only found in developing countries; it is in fact found more commonly in the Western world where people are eating foods with no nutrient value to them whatsoever but use calorie counting in an effort to stay slim – it is crazy!

The Truth: Restriction Never Works

As a coach, one of the key points I teach the women I'm working with is that restriction does not work. On a physiological level, when we restrict the food source to our bodies, they will simply hold on to as much energy as possible in order to survive. As a result, you will not lose weight.

If you consider the body as a machine that you live in, and look at it from a functional perspective, you realise that its job is to keep you alive. There are a million different mechanisms at work every minute of every day, on an autonomic level, attempting to fulfil that purpose. No wonder it's storing up energy when you stop feeding it! To think that we can trick it, overcome it, or defy scientific laws and get what we want by bargaining with it, is doing it a disservice.

Yes, with complete restriction, you would ultimately lose weight. However, maintaining this level of restriction is not possible because it goes against the limbic need to survive. If you are starving yourself and there is food accessible to you then the urge to resist will be too great - your body and your brain's survival instincts will kick in. This urge is your survival mechanism saying, "I've got to have energy."

We're not designed to starve. Our body produces a hormone called ghrelin, the hunger hormone, that takes over at a certain point. This is as true now as it was when we first evolved. When our ancestors were hungry, this hormone would tell them, "Go and forage. Go and find food. Go and eat." We abide by the same science, the same hormones, the same rules.

Balancing your blood sugar is one of the most important things that you can do when it comes to weight loss, gaining energy, and smashing cravings. When your blood sugar is all over the place, you're much more prone to mood swings, hormonal imbalances, and cravings. If you're eating sugar to compensate, this prompts your body to release more adrenaline, creating a self-fulfilling cycle. Plus, once you start eating sugar, you crave even more sugar – it becomes quite addictive. And the side effects are terrible. I run sugar-free weeks in my group programs and I've seen people go through dreadful headaches, sweats, and fevers. It can be a full on withdrawal process.

Most women beat themselves up for not being able to fight cravings when actually it is simply their body releasing ghrelin because they are not satiated. It is amazing how many people find their cravings completely disappear when they start eating enough fibre and guess what – they lose weight easily!

When the mind feels restricted, when there is something that you're not allowed to have or not allowed to do, you're going to be constantly thinking about that thing. So, if the belief is that you can have anything that nurtures and makes you feel good, guess what? The intense desire or need for that forbidden food is gone because you can have it without judgement. Once you eliminate the restriction and the punishment, you negate the need to "cheat" and break free from the cycle entirely.

There are many reasons why diets don't work. Our bodies aren't made to sustain long-term significant weight loss and, more often than not, it's not even in our best interest. Dieting defies the intuition that our bodies have developed over centuries of evolution. We are designed to be healthy and to be well. As soon as we start to restrict calories, it sets off alarm bells in our body. Our systems panic and slow down. We start to burn muscle and instead we hold on to fat, which will keep us alive for longer. I'm talking about a full blown change in our metabolism. And the less lean mass that we have, the fewer calories that we burn.

Ultimately, dieting makes us fatter in the long run. Ironic, right? In fact, 60% of people who are dieting put more weight back on than what they lost. They've messed with their metabolism. Dieting trains your brain to make food harder to resist. It's a survival mechanism.

Remember, your body is amazing and it wants to survive at all costs! We need to eat to live. Calories are converted into energy, and we exist off that energy. Without it, our bodies will start to shut down. When food is in short supply, our hormones will kick in to convince you to eat. And those are much, much harder to ignore when you have been dieting for long periods of time. When you deprive yourself of certain foods, you start to crave them. Your brain seeks out the foods it hasn't been allowed.

This is why we get so caught up in the cycle of dieting. Dieting messes with your hunger and satisfaction cues. We diet, and then we lose weight, but then we put it back on because we go back to eating normally – only this time, we put on even more weight than we did before. It's what happens when you mess with your metabolism. Fundamentally, restricting calories is not a sensible thing to do when it comes to weight loss.

Myth: Calories In, Calories Out Is All That Matters

This myth is two-fold. It tells us that all calories are equal, and you will lose weight as long as you are keeping track of the total calories you've consumed - no matter what the nutritional value of the food. "I ate three Mars bars, but that's still within my calorie quota."

The second aspect of this myth is that you can exercise off a bad diet. "It doesn't matter if I over-ate, I'll burn it off at the gym tomorrow."

Truth: Calories Are Old School, Nutrients Are Now Cool

To reduce your body to such a simplistic rule is to do a real disservice – to both yourself and the incredible machine that you live in. Food can't be quantified in a single number. It's not like adding up your daily step count. The quality of what you're eating – the nutritional value of your food – is so important. It impacts how your body utilises that energy. Take, for example, 200 calories of avocado (banned at Weight Watchers) and 200 calories of chocolate. The nutrient-dense avocado is going to behave very differently inside the body compared to the simple processed carbohydrates of the chocolate.

Instead of calculating your calorie net worth, ask yourself, "How can I nurture my body with the nutrients that it needs, and fuel it with the energy it requires, so that I feel good?"

This extends to exercise and movement. This also should be a way to nourish yourself, not to sweat out calories from over-doing it the day before. That mentality is punishment for the body, mind and soul. Absolutely everything is about you feeling good.

Movement and food are simply ways to stoke your life force, or your essence. In Chinese medicine this is known as the Qi. Qi runs through energy channels, called meridians, in the body. When Qi becomes blocked, or stagnant, then the body becomes weak or heavy. When we don't

179

look after ourselves, when we punish ourselves through improper nutrition and lack of movement, then our energy is depleted, and our life force diminishes.

Nourishment provides you with the energy to thrive. Your body is to be celebrated, loved and cherished through every action you take, and every thought you have.

Myth: Willpower Is a Thing

A truly dangerous myth is that the reason you can't lose weight is because you lack the willpower to do so. If you think that you can't lose weight because you can't stick to a diet then right away, you are setting yourself up to fail! You're starting your journey to health with "I can't" and "I'm not enough." You are starting your journey with hate and negative energy towards yourself, by immediately questioning your power as a woman and as a human.

This is not a reflection of your personality or your perceived inability. This is about what the body can do on a physiological level - the rules that govern us by science.

Remember that your body is trying to keep you alive because it loves you. It wants you to be healthy, and it wants you to feel good. That's the body's intention and purpose. Yet most of us don't have any real relationship with our bodies, which feel disconnected from us. Instead, we say things like, "I hate my body. It doesn't work for me. It's ugly. I hate it."

Truth: Willpower Is Not a Thing

When we are hungry or when we're stressed, our body releases hormones to tell us to eat. There's no amount of willpower that will ever overcome that.

We have approximately 130,000 calories of fat storage and 2,500 calories of glycogen storage in the body. When we're stressed and we're in a state of fight or flight, we pull from our glycogen store - which has a total reserve of our average daily calorie expenditure. So, if you've been stressed all day, by the time the afternoon rolls around your body will be about two-thirds of the way through that glycogen store. At this point, it will start to make demands: "I need to eat something." That's why women often find it really easy to eat well in the morning but by 3pm, they've gone and raided the chocolate stash. The body is looking for something that can be rapidly absorbed and converted into energy, so these snack cravings will almost always be simple carbohydrates. It's telling you that its inbuilt survival mechanism – the one that stores up energy so you can run away in the event of danger – is running on empty, and you need to fuel up fast. When we're stressed, the process of turning fat into energy is too slow; the body is looking for an immediate hit instead.

We can't separate our body out into parts and try to treat the symptoms individually. The thoughts that we're having, the information that we're reading…all of this impacts the relationship we have with ourselves, and the food choices that we're making.

Why do I crave something sweet when I have just eaten?

I get asked this question ALL the time! Do you crave something sweet after eating, even if you are full?

The reason you crave something sweet when you have just eaten is because digestion takes such a huge amount of energy. In fact, digestion uses more energy than any other process in your body. If you have just eaten a heavy meal or simply eaten too much, your body will release a hormone (good old ghrelin again) to tell you it needs some energy to be able to complete the enormous task it has in front of it, which is to convert all of the food you have just eaten and turn it into components your body actually needs.

Isn't your body incredible?! When we start to understand why it does what it does and that it is not about our fault or inability to achieve something we can let go of these stories and start working with her. She is amazing, this body of yours; it is time to honour her, respect her and nourish her in the way she longs for you to.

To overcome this, here are a few things you can do. Try eating until you are 80% full rather than eating everything on your plate. I know you have probably been taught to clear your plate but fortunately we are a couple of generations on from being post war now. We can leave food behind. I know you might not like wasting food but that doesn't mean you need to eat it. (How many times have you started a diet only after you have eaten all the Christmas chocolates to get them out of the house?) Use leftovers for lunch the next day, and start buying and cooking smaller amounts. You do not have to eat food to avoid wasting it.

Dieting teaches you that you can't trust your own body's wisdom. It tells you what to eat and how much. But how can anyone know your body and how it feels better than you? You can trust your body. You can trust how you feel. Healing requires you to awaken the conscious relationship you have with your body.

Bringing consciousness into your relationship with food and your body is an essential part of the healing journey. How often do you eat in a rush or eat whilst you are doing something else? Ask yourself questions when you are eating. What does hungry feel like to you? What does full feel like? What does it feel like to leave some food on your plate?

Nourishing your body is a sacred practice. Instead of rushing through cooking and eating and thinking of it as a chore, imagine it being part of your self-care. Bring presence and joy to the process. You are giving your body healing nourishment. Slow down and make space for it. Taste your food and chew it properly, enjoying the flavours. Put your phone away, sit at a table and turn off the TV. Simply be present with yourself and your meal. Think about each bite of food nourishing each of the 50 trillion cells that make you who you are.

If you are honest, how regularly do you make eating a sacred practice? It is not something we have been taught to do, is it?

Slow down. Listen. Your body knows the answers. Your head will tell you it doesn't but your body and soul know. You need to make space to hear.

Below are a few more concepts and tips to help you transform the way you eat without feeling like you are on a restrictive diet.

Crowding Out

Rather than taking an all or nothing route, simply focus on getting some good things into your body. Perhaps start your day with a smoothie that includes broccoli, spinach, blueberries and banana. (I know that sounds gross but it is really not. I can't tell you how quickly it becomes the favourite recipe of the women I work with, once they get over the "really Anna, that is too far" hurdle!)

Crowding out is the concept of filling your body with lots of good stuff it loves. It is not saying no to the things which are tempting; it is simply about bringing balance to the way you eat on a daily basis. Rather than thinking that you have ruined everything if you eat something which doesn't feel healthy, put the guilt down and eat something healthy and nourishing as well. Give your body what it needs to help it process the less healthy foods.

The 80 / 20 Rule

Aim to eat fruit and vegetables 80% of the time. When I say fruit and vegetables, I also mean legumes, beans, and wholegrains to keep you full. If you eat these things 80% of the time and 20% of the time you are eating things that perhaps have less nutritional value, you are doing great.

The Mind Diet

There are a few books that have been life-changing for me when it comes to food and I recommend you read them too.

- The China Study – Colin T Campbell

- How Not to Die – Michael Greger

- The Starch Solution – John McDougall

- The Food Revolution – John Robbins

- The Mind Diet – Maggie Moon

The Mind Diet suggests foods you need to be aiming for on a daily / weekly basis – I believe this is a great rule of thumb to guide you:

- Green, leafy vegetables: Aim for six or more servings per week. This includes kale, spinach, cooked greens and salads.

- All other vegetables: Try to eat plenty of other vegetables in addition to the green leafy vegetables at least once a day. A raw salad once a day with plenty of colours is a really great addition.

- Berries: Eat berries at least twice a week. Although the published research only includes strawberries, you should also consume other berries like blueberries, raspberries and blackberries for their antioxidant benefits.

- Nuts: Try to get five servings of nuts or more each week.

- Olive oil: Use olive oil as your main cooking oil. Use cold pressed, organic, extra virgin oil and use it sparingly.

- Whole grains: Aim for at least one serving daily. Choose whole grains like oatmeal, quinoa, brown rice, and whole-wheat pasta.

- Beans: Include beans in at least four meals every week. This includes all beans, lentils and soybeans.

- Wine: Aim for no more than one glass daily. Both red and white wine may benefit the brain and research suggests a little wine actually helps you live longer. However, alcohol is also a depressant and causes anxiety. There is also a heavy correlation between some cancers and alcohol, so you need to tune into your body and how you feel about alcohol personally. It is a poison, after all. I know I feel better when I don't drink!

Stay Hydrated

I don't need to tell you how important it is to stay hydrated for your health, weight management, energy, hormone balance, immune system – basically everything in your body. But how good are you at remembering?! I carry a 1-litre water bottle with me wherever I go and I fill it up twice a day. A great rule of thumb is to divide your weight in kilos by 30 and that is how many litres you need to drink.

Think. Feel. Act.

As soon as I start a diet, I start eating! Sound familiar? Of course you do! You are taking away the one thing you have allowed yourself for pleasure. There is a part of you screaming so desperately to be seen and loved, expressing that she is HUNGRY! Take away the only thing that helps you feel full and she will shout louder.

Your mind is designed to move away from pain and towards pleasure. It creates habit loops to help you feel into higher vibration moods if a thought has taken you down to a low place.. Food is often used in a habit loop because we release dopamine when we eat. All of this happens without you thinking about it – your body is working to make sure you feel happy.

You have a thought. You judge it and it impacts your feelings. Your mind releases an action to help you feel better.

Often you will end up eating without knowing what happened.

That is why understanding how you talk to yourself matters. If you are talking to yourself negatively then it is highly likely your mind will be trying to find a way to lift your mood. Take a moment to shift, getting into a state of appreciation or changing your perspective.

Affirmation

- When I experience low mood feelings, I take time to get into a state of appreciation before allowing the old habit of food to kick back in

Exercise

Changing your diet is hands down one of the most transformative things you could ever do for yourself and your body. Bringing consciousness to your eating is one of the most powerful steps along your healing journey. Asking yourself questions will help you understand your patterns more deeply and in turn, help you create changes which serve instead of sabotage.

The Anna Anderson HEAL™ method is an acronym I created to help you break patterns and build awareness. You can stick it on your fridge or the cupboards in your kitchen to remind you. If you catch yourself sniffing around the kitchen, slow down, take a breath and use these questions to create some space and build awareness around a desired behaviour which serves you.

The *H* stands for *hungry*. Am I actually hungry? Why am I about to eat? What am I truly hungry for that is not food?

The *E* stands for *emotion*. What emotion am I experiencing right now?

The *A* stands for *alternative*. Is there an alternative? Is there something else that I could eat which is more nourishing? Is there something else I could do right now which would feel nurturing and loving?

The *L* stands for *love*. What would love for myself look like instead? Is there something else I could do? What loving action could I take? What do I really need?

The Truth About Self-Care

Let's summarise what you have actioned so far. You have gotten clear on what you DO want. You now understand that there is a part of you who is not being honoured, and started learning about the hungry feminine energy with you. The next step is to start to honour her.

The answer always starts with self-care and awareness.

The movement toward self-love and self-care is fantastic, but if we don't truly understand what self-care is, then it doesn't really help. Sure, self-care can be the external stuff: getting your hair done, painting your nails, or getting a massage. Those things are nice but they have to come along with the deep internal work too: learning who you are, making space for you in your life, meditation, connecting to your breath, reprogramming limiting beliefs, and unpacking suppressed emotions.

One of my clients, Rachel, told me she was so relieved to hear that self-care wasn't about getting her hair done because whenever she went to spend time on herself in this way it didn't make her feel any better. She thought there was something wrong with her!

Real self-care is learning to love yourself unconditionally. It is learning to identify, listen to, and honour your inner calling. Learning to be kind to the incredible human that you are. Learning to love the body you live in and to nourish it so that it can thrive for you and support you in living your best life. When your body feels good, and you have energy and a clear head – life is way more joyful. Happiness is found within you. It is not a condition based on external factors. If you are basing your happiness on things outside of yourself then it is conditional and out of your control. Your joy and happiness are found in deep love and acceptance of who you are.

Right now, you are probably thinking at some deep, unconscious level that you are only worthy of achieving or having the life you desire when you have lost weight.

Yet that simply isn't true. You are worthy now and this elephant in the room has been keeping you in a holding pattern for years.

You are worthy. You are good enough.

What if you could have everything exactly how you want it? What if we simply drop this whole focus on weight loss and instead make it about your health, about feeling good, about having energy, and liberating yourself from these shackles so that you can live a life of freedom and joy? Because that life is waiting for you.

I love this Taoist teaching that reminds us to relax and let life flow:

> When an old farmer's stallion won a prize at a country show, his neighbour called round to congratulate him. The old farmer said, "Who knows what is good and what is bad?"
>
> The next day some thieves came and stole the valuable animal. When the neighbour came to commiserate with him, the old man replied, "Who knows what is good and what is bad?"
>
> A few days later the spirited stallion escaped from the thieves and joined a herd of wild mares, leading them back to the farm. The neighbour called in to share the farmer's joy, but the farmer responded, "Who knows what is good and what is bad?"
>
> The following day, while trying to break in one of the mares, the farmer's son got thrown and fractured his leg. The neighbour called to share the farmer's sorrow, but the old man's attitude remained the same as before.
>
> The following week the army passed by, forcibly conscripting soldiers for the war, but they did not take the farmer's son because he couldn't walk. And the neighbour thought to himself, "Who knows what is good and what is bad?" realising that the old farmer must be a Taoist sage.

"Imagine the woman you want to be. Think of what her daily life, her habits, and routines would be. Start showing up to those habits and routines, start building them, step by step and day by day. You don't become her like magic. You build her. Start building." – Jamie Varon

Whatever areas you decide to work on, know this: you get one shot at this journey called life. Life isn't just about the big moments that we are waiting and searching for. It is in the joy and simplicity of every day. You create joy by looking around you and noticing how wonderful your life actually is. And if there are things you want to change then that is OK, you can do that too! It starts with appreciating what you already have, including that incredible body of yours - because quite frankly, if you didn't have it, you wouldn't be here.

It is time to change, sister. It is time to love yourself and your life and take action every day towards the truth of who you are. You are only stuck if you believe you are.

"Most people miss their whole lives, you know. Listen, life isn't when you are standing on top of a mountain looking at the sunset. Life isn't waiting at the altar or the moment your child is born or that time you were swimming in deep water and a dolphin came up alongside you. These are fragments. 10 or 12 grains of sand spread throughout your entire existence. They are not life. Life is brushing your teeth or making a sandwich or watching the news or waiting for a bus. Or walking. Every day, thousands of tiny events happen and if you are not watching, if you're careful, if you don't capture

them and make them COUNT, you could miss it. You could miss your whole life." – Toni Jordan

Non-Negotiable Rituals

As you move through all of these ideas you might start to feel overwhelmed with a big, long list of all the things you have to do! That is not what we are looking for; remember, this is all about feeling good and making decisions from a place of empowerment and self-worth.

Creating new habits takes time and consistency. Be gentle with yourself, take regular steady steps to create routines that serve deeper self-awareness and self-care. Go back to your Wheel of Life areas of focus and think about what next step you would like to take to move forward. What one thing do you most want to focus on in your life? Chunking goals down into bite-sized and manageable steps is key.

As you build your foundations of self-care you will find practices that serve you deeply. I call these rituals. They are sacred acts of nourishment and care for yourself that are essential to your wellbeing. As you build upon your steps, I suggest you create daily habits that serve your bigger picture – things you do every day and become your non-negotiable rituals.

This might look like getting up a little earlier in the morning to make space for quiet reflection and meditation, practising yoga or breath-work, or replacing your daily glass of wine with a glass of kombucha – it is up to you! These sacred rituals become your new habits. Things you do, even when you don't feel it – they just become your new normal.

I am a true early bird, I love to get up in the morning and take time for myself before everyone else wakes up. It has become a non-negotiable for me to practice yoga for 20 minutes, followed by meditation and appreciation. I also used to have an evening habit of snacking on the sofa, but by creating a new non-negotiable of 10 minutes' meditation before sitting down, I now find it much easier to make conscious choices.

Creating rituals from a new identity is an incredibly powerful thing to do. When you create a habit from a place of 'not-enoughness' then it is highly likely it will fly out the window after a few days. But if you create your new identity first (go back to the letter you wrote from your future self) and start there, you are much more likely to keep up your new habits. What would that version of you do? What non-negotiable rituals would she have? Set up your rituals from your new identity and they will feel empowering instead of like a punishment.

Affirmations

- I accept and love myself, exactly as I am

- I nourish my mind and body with healthy food and thought

- I am excited about how my day might unfold

- My mind is at peace. My body is at ease

- Every day I become stronger and healthier

- I am patient, kind and forgiving

- I think positive, loving and empowering thoughts

- I believe in myself, truly and deeply

- I am powerfully courageous

- I do not let feelings of fear of doubt stand in the way of my greatness

- I know there is always a solution to any problem

Exercise

Answer these questions in your journal:

- What does self-care truly mean to me?

- How am I feeling right now on a scale of 1-10? What is impacting that feeling?

- What form of self-care do I need to work on this month (a habit, a boundary, mindset etc)?

- What lesson have I learned about myself in the last month?

- How is my sleep and bedtime routine? How could I improve it?

- What am I looking forward to?

Here are self-care rituals you might like to introduce in your life. See which ones you connect to and start to implement them into your life on a regular basis:

- Go for a walk in nature

- Drink two litres of water

- Eat an extra serving of fruit or vegetables

- Unfollow something on social media that doesn't feel good

- Talk to your partner or friend about your needs and how they might support you

- Write in your journal for 10 minutes

- Connect with your breath

- Take a night off alcohol (or a week, or a month!)

- Declutter a cupboard

- Have a bath

- Grab an adult colouring book or paint, draw or create in a way you love

- Read a book

- Practice yoga

- Listen to your favourite song

- Take a shower and moisturise

- Write down five things you love about yourself

- Check out your finances and set up a little saving pot – even if you simply save a penny a day, you are saving!

- Ask for help

- Say no to something

- Go to the cinema on your own

- Stop the scroll – take a day off social media

- Have a nap

- Cuddle your pet or favourite human

- Go to bed 15 minutes earlier than usual

- Cook your favourite meal and slow down whilst you eat it. Taste the flavour and imagine how it is nourishing your body as you eat

Stop and Listen

That leads me into consciousness. How much quiet do you have in your life? How much time do you spend doing nothing? The answer to finding out who you are and what you need is found in peace. It is found in time spent alone in deep internal enquiry. Become your own best friend: listen, tune into what your inner voice is saying about what you need, what your body is saying about what you need. Create enough quiet space in your life to be able to hear yourself.

I remember when I started this journey, I was terrified of the quiet. I always had the TV or radio on in the background. I couldn't sit still without my phone. If I was eating alone, I was scrolling on social media as well. I was living a very unconscious life. Quite frankly, I just didn't like myself very much. If I sat with myself, I was either bored or frightened of where my mind would go – it was too painful to experience all the emotions, so I pushed them down, ignored them, kept busy and used food and alcohol to numb them.

But guess what – that doesn't work! They are all there, sitting in our subconscious, playing out like a broken record until we slow down and take a look at them.

Awareness is curative. My coach has hammered that statement into my mind again and again and again. It is in awareness that we find out who we are. We build a relationship with ourselves by slowing down and listening to our own needs. If you were in a relationship with anyone else and you completely ignored them all of the time, paid them no attention, and were in actual fact, cruel to them – telling them how ugly they were, how incapable they were, judging and criticising them – how would they feel? The relationship probably wouldn't last long.

That is what you are doing to yourself every day. Those unkind voices are not serving you and in fact they are not true. There is no way you would talk to anyone else the way you talk to yourself. It is time to slow down and make some space for yourself so that you can start to pick apart what is fact and what is fiction in your mind.

The truth of who you are is love. Anything else is simply a pattern you have been playing out, keeping you stuck. Nourish yourself the way you would a child. Listen to yourself. Be kind.

Busy doesn't mean worthy.

We have been taught since we were little girls that our worth is in busyness and serving others. The reality is, you serve others when your cup is full. Your own self-care and nourishment is what heals the world. If you want the world to be different, start with yourself and light the way for others from there. From a full cup, you can truly act from a place of service.

Affirmations

- I enjoy taking the time to simply be

- I make the conscious choice to slow down

- I enjoy the journey

- I make time to observe life

- My wellbeing and joy comes from a place of peace within me

Exercise

Meditation is one of the most powerful forms of self-care and transformation you can practice. It is the first thing any spiritual teacher recommends as a self-development practice because it takes you out of egoic thinking and connects you to the truth of who you are.

Lots of times people tell me "Oh, I can't meditate – it doesn't work for me." When I ask them why, they say it either didn't work or they can't quieten their head. The secret is to get out of Beta brain waves (busy thoughts and doing energy) and into Alpha brain waves (the quiet knowing within you).

My top tip for meditation and shifting between these two states is to imagine feeling unconditional love. Close your eyes and do it now. It doesn't matter if you have never felt that from a person – imagine what it would feel like. A warm, safe and glowy feeling, right? That is changing your state and that is the place you want to meditate from.

The truth about meditation is that it's a practice. You need to be consistent with it, otherwise you will not experience the benefits. The other truth about meditation is you must let go of the goal of quieting your head – in fact, you have to completely let go of any goal. The purpose of meditation is to simply be. Use the exercise above to get into a different state and be there as much as you can.

Set the intention to meditate every day for 10-15 minutes for 30 days. Be specific about a time you are going to do it, get clear on the space where you are going to sit, and make sure it is the same each time. Use an anchor to ground and prepare you before your practice. Perhaps you light a candle, read a favourite piece of text that moves you, or pull an oracle card – whatever works for you. Just be consistent about this being your time to connect to your breath and slow down.

You can use guided meditations, which are great if you are starting out, but I do suggest meditating in silence and on your own if you can. Set a timer and sit and connect with your breath. Follow your breath in and out, breathing down to your tummy. Don't worry about silencing your thoughts, just become an observer of them. Use your breath as your guide and if your mind wanders off, that is absolutely OK. As soon as you notice, gently bring your focus back to your breath. Don't get frustrated or be unkind to yourself – simply guide yourself back.

You might have moments of silence in your head or you might have none at all – it doesn't matter. Over time, as you practice, your experience will change. Your job is simply to be with whatever comes up, not to judge it.

If you notice noise around you, let it be there. See if you can notice being surrounded by sounds and sensations but not thinking about them, simply being with your breath.

You will need to be disciplined about this practice, which is why it is a good idea to do it for 30 days straight and then review.

See how you get on and notice the difference it makes! It truly is a wonderful practice. Enjoy!

You Are Your Top Priority

I hope by now we are making some great progress and you are experiencing some great breakthroughs. Let's take a look at self-care, but first – let me bust a really common little myth.

Myth: It's Selfish to Put Yourself First

The more I do, the more successful I am. Right? There's a masculinity in proving your worth; in being enough, earning enough, and having enough. In response, we women tend to hold a deeply ingrained belief that it is selfish to put ourselves first.

Truth: Everything Around You Is Better When You Are Full First

"But it's selfish if I put myself first!" I hear this all the time. Actually, this is the *least* selfish thing you can do. It's selfless because when you're full, everyone else is better off for it too. When a woman is full from the inside out, everybody around her benefits. She will parent better; she won't be shouting at everyone because she's not low on energy and she's not beating herself up because of what she just ate. Her blood sugar will be balanced. She's had time for herself. As a result, every relationship in her life will be better.

Everyone wants you – as the nurturer, as the divine feminine, as the heart of your family or community – to be in a good place. The light that you carry will radiate out to everybody around you. That is your responsibility.

If we take the time and do the work to focus on ourselves, this positive energy manifests all through our lives. When we fail to put ourselves first, this will show up and contaminate all areas of life too. This comes through in behaviours like shouting at the kids, not having sex, being unhappy in your relationship, not honouring the stuff that is actually true, and hating what you see in the mirror every day. The more we are giving, giving, giving – because we think our worth is in what we do for everybody else – the more we are depleting our own energy.

It's up to you to keep your cup full. There are energy fillers that keep you topped up and energy drillers that drain you. We all have certain things that naturally fill us up, and others that make us feel rubbish. These are the choices that we make, the people we spend time with, the foods we eat, and the things we do.

Yet it almost feels unnatural for many women to feel comfortable with receiving. We're taught to give all the time. To receive money, to receive sexual pleasure, to receive anything as a woman has an ancestral taboo around it. Sex is bad. To enjoy your body is bad. To gain pleasure from sex is bad. Even the simple act of receiving a compliment feels incredibly hard for some of us. Have you ever said "Oh, I got it in the sale" or "This old thing?" when someone compliments what you are wearing? I used to do it all of the time. Simply saying thank you somehow felt unnatural or wrong.

All this is the result of incredibly deep societal conditioning. It's uncomfortable to think that you're worthy of having, of receiving, of prioritising yourself. To accept these is to fight a pattern you've been living with forever. When you receive something, that is not the time to question your worth – it's the time to confirm it.

So many women go through life with an underlying current of not feeling like we are worth our own time. This is all wrapped up in the belief that spending time on yourself is selfish. But where is all your time actually going?

The Johari Window is a coaching tool with four time quadrants that can help you organise your thoughts and recognise your time priorities and behavioural patterns.

1. The urgent and important

2. Not urgent but still important

3. Urgent but not important

4. Not urgent and not important

You now fit under URGENT AND IMPORTANT! Feel good now. Be happy now. Enjoy life now. Take care of yourself now.

We react immediately to things that we think are urgent, like work or our children. We put the not urgent but still important things, like our relationship with ourselves, our partners, or our health, to the side. We spend our time on the not urgent and not important – scrolling on social media, binging on Netflix and wasting time because we don't feel fulfilled within.

Do you have time to be sick? Do you have time to spend feeling the way that you are? Is this bringing you joy? Do you want to spend the last few decades of your life living this way? Do you have time for that? What are you prepared to put up with, and where are you prepared to compromise?

If we are serious about self-care, then we prioritise ourselves – and we find that in fact, we actually always have the time to do so. If we let go of the not urgent and the not important, we free up time for ourselves. It's about slowing down and releasing the idea that our potential is in being a human being, not a human doing.

Affirmations

- I take time to prioritise my needs on a daily basis
- I nourish myself in ways which feel good
- I slow down and listen to my intuition
- It feels good to practice self-care

Exercise

Below are some examples of ways you can make more space and peace in your life. Implement some or all of these things to help you slow down and prioritise yourself:

- Turn your notifications off on your phone

- Leave your phone downstairs when you go to bed (don't use your phone as an alarm – buy one of those old-fashioned alarm clocks!)

- Eat away from your desk and without your phone

- Practice driving without the radio on (music is fun too, just explore the quiet sometimes!)

- Stop listening to the (bad) news in the morning

- Walk in nature for 30 minutes by yourself

- Spend time on your own

- Go out for food by yourself and leave your phone at home

- Sit quietly and observe your breath

- Read instead of watching TV

Who Are You Really?

"Knowing yourself is the beginning of all wisdom."
- Aristotle

Behind every behaviour there is always a need. If rather than judging and criticising your behaviour, you instead explore the need behind it, you can start to detect patterns and replace them with others that serve you more deeply.

Your job is to honour yourself and learn how to nurture and nourish all that you are. Remember, you are a goddess. Allow her to be uncovered and expressed. There are parts of you that you've kept pushed down and hidden for so long. Food is a comfort to the true hunger you feel. The hunger to be seen, to be heard, to realise your potential, to laugh, adventure and be playful, to express your inner wild.

The more we battle to look a certain way, the more unloved we feel and the more we seek comfort. This is an invitation to explore yourself and your needs.

Who am I?

Have you ever asked yourself that question? Or perhaps you feel like you really don't know who you are?

Often I hear this from women who get in touch with me when their children are getting more independent or leaving home. All of a sudden they find they have space to explore the bigger questions life throws at us. In my opinion, this is exciting! It means you are ready to explore the wonderful and delicious truth of who you are.

As I mentioned earlier, when I had my son, I felt I had lost my identity. I had zero idea who I was anymore. In actual fact, I had never really known who I was because I had based my entire identity in things outside of myself. So when my life changed dramatically, I lost those things, and it felt like I lost myself. It happened again when I gave up my job. I felt like I had lost my identity – the one "respectable" thing I had left to hold onto as a single mother. Of course, this couldn't be further from the truth, but part of me felt that giving up my job meant I had failed or become a statistic.

What I now know to be true, and would have loved to have known back then, is you are not any of the roles you play. Your identity is not mother, grandmother, wife, sister, friend, daughter, or your job title. Whilst we tend to judge and compare ourselves based on what we have and what we do, that's not what defines us. For example, if you wanted, you could fly a plane. You simply haven't learned yet (or maybe you have!) so therefore limiting your identity to a skill you have or haven't yet learned is restrictive. With that mindset you will consistently look for the things you have not achieved and your world will get smaller and smaller. If you focus on all the times you have tried and failed to lose weight, you build deep seated beliefs that you cannot create what you desire in life. That becomes your story and, if you are not careful, your identity.

Who you actually are is joy, love, and light. Your true self is joyful, playful, relaxed, and happy. She is delicious and sensuous. She delights in her body, she delights in nature, she dances, she laughs, she wears her hair messy, she does not care what she looks like because she knows she is beautiful, she connects to her intuition, and she walks barefoot with the Earth. You are a soul who is expansive beyond measure. The only thing that limits you is the constraints of your mind.

Your identity and purpose is found in getting out of your head and moving into your heart and soul. Your purpose is the expansion of your soul. You know who you are. Your head might say you don't, but your heart does. All the answers you seek are within you. You will find yourself in the quiet space you create.

When you allow yourself to be in a state of blissful contentment without the external pressures or expectations of your mind and the limits of your belief system your purpose will become extremely clear. You will find meaning in everything you do. Your identity and purpose are found in you following your bliss.

When you know who you are, you will have less internal conflict and a deeper sense of confidence. You can set boundaries and you will feel less pressured by others. From a sense of knowing, you can make decisions that serve you and that in turn will lead to more happiness, self-love, and acceptance.

Knowing your values will help you understand how you can move through life honouring yourself at a deep level, matching up your identity with how you show up in the external world. Values are the things you hold most dear in your life. They are what you prioritise over anything else and whether you are aware of them or not, they will be a driving force behind the decisions you make.

Sometimes our values might conflict – like family and freedom. Sometimes we might be living out of alignment with our values, for example, doing a job that doesn't really align with who we are. Doing something outside of your values will rarely make you feel good and will, most likely, exhaust you.

It's OK to have conflicting values. The important thing is making sure you are honouring all parts of yourself. If you value freedom but you have children – how do you make space for yourself, and how do you have fun? Think about how you can implement freedom in your new life (without feeling guilty). Perhaps going away for a weekend once in a while, or seeing a friend without your children in tow, is going to help you feel more aligned and connected to who you are. Remember, you have permission to honour your needs. Your family will experience a grounded and happier version of you when you honour your needs, so there really is no need for guilt when you take care of yourself.

The exercise in this section will guide you through how to elicit your values.

Get to know yourself as you would a friend.

Ask yourself questions.

Meet your own needs.

Build a relationship with yourself and fall in love with who you are.

Setting Boundaries

As you start to better understand who you are, you can draw a ring of loving fire around yourself.

Are you a people pleaser? Because I promise you that is not doing your health or weight any good. If you are busy running around trying to keep everyone happy and dishonouring yourself, of course you are going to seek comfort.

Self-care is not always easy; we have established that. It is about breaking through beliefs and conditioning, learning to meet your needs and talk to yourself in loving ways. It is about gently making space to listen to your heart and take action towards what you need rather than what you think you 'should' do or what someone else needs.

I believe one of the most important parts of self-care is showing up for yourself and doing uncomfortable things that you do not always want to do. In other words – boundaries!

Boundaries are tough for most of us. Due to my need to be loved and accepted, I found it very hard to say no to other people. But as I learned to love myself, I didn't need to receive approval from others any more in order to validate myself and guess what?! That made me more likeable to those I liked to spend time with. The people who I didn't align with fell away. And that is OK. Not everyone is going to like you. That is not a bad thing! What you think of you matters more than anything else and the more you vibrate with loving energy for the glorious feminine being that you are, the more you will attract your tribe. You do not need to please others to be enough or to be loveable.

There were so many times in life I put up with something that was 100% unacceptable because I was too scared to say that it wasn't OK. Through my work, I have seen this to be true for many others too. You have permission to say no.

"Boundaries are a part of self-care. They are healthy, normal, and necessary." – Doreen Virtue

*E*very time you say yes to someone, when you really want to say no, you are saying no to yourself. That has to stop. It is absolutely not your responsibility to keep everyone else happy.

Moving forward, get curious. Is there a belief in there that is keeping you stuck? What is the reason behind why you are saying yes to things? Why do you need to make others happy before yourself? Deep down, do you feel loveable? Do you know you are already enough? Remember that beauty lies within you; the only person who truly needs to accept you is yourself. From that deep place of knowing and love for yourself – you will bloom as you are meant to.

Setting boundaries is something you will get better and better at as you practice. Practice setting boundaries every day. Set healthy boundaries with your children, your friends, your family, at work, and with your partner. If you don't want to do something, say no.

You need to stop spending time with people who don't make you feel good and you need to communicate effectively what you want. I am not saying for one minute this is easy. I have had to have some really uncomfortable conversations with people to explain how I am feeling or that I don't want to do something. But the truth is, even though it was uncomfortable – it was my truth and therefore doing so was about serving myself rather than giving myself away.

If you dread being around someone and each time you come away afterwards feeling awful, it is not kind to the other person to keep going this way. In trying to be kind and keep other people happy, you are actually being unkind to yourself and the other person. If you are truly, painfully honest, it is because you are frightened of having an uncomfortable conversation and hurting them. And if you are even more painfully honest, it is not even about hurting them – it is that YOU don't want to feel the discomfort of hurting them. Time to pull your big girl pants up my love – it is time to put those boundaries in place and start honouring yourself.

Boundaries do not mean being rude, not in the slightest. They mean putting a loving and gentle boundary around your energy and making sure you honour yourself first. Boundaries can be set with love, kindness and grace. 'No' can be said in the most loving way. Examples of ways to start practising your boundary setting include:

- Saying no

- Expecting respect

- Explaining how you feel

- Asking for space

- Communicating your needs

- Setting boundaries with time – when are you working, when are you resting?

- Asking for help

Being an Empath

There are whole books written on just this topic, so I simply want to make you aware in case this is not something you have heard of before; it will absolutely impact your relationship with food if you aren't using this superpower in a skillful way.

An empath is someone who *feels* other people's feelings. Many women who come to work with me are empaths who never realised it. Imagine that you are energy, and you walk around in your own sphere of energy – like a golden orb of light surrounding you.

Signs of being an empath include:

- You take on other people's emotions as your own
- Sometimes you experience sudden overwhelming emotion in public
- You can read how someone is feeling without them saying anything
- The vibe in the room matters to you
- You can always understand where someone is coming from.
- Tragic or violent events on TV impact you greatly
- You cannot see someone in pain without wanting to help
- Your mood can go from high to low at the drop of a hat

Being an empath means you are highly sensitive to other people's energy fields as well as your own. You are most likely in a caring profession because of your ability to sense how people feel but you may also find it very difficult to set boundaries. You can read a room, you are highly intuitive, you will know things without knowing how or why – it is just a feeling. When you spend time with people, their energy bleeds into your energy field, which means you are often carrying around other people's energy rather than your own. You might not understand the reason behind your feelings or why life can feel so hard, or why you seem to go from feeling very high to very low so easily.

It is not only other people who impact you. You will carry around the energy of the news, the TV shows you watch, what you read – everything you surround yourself with. It can be exhausting.

As Napoleon Hill said, "Imagine there is an energy constantly flowing to, with and through you; this energy is also flowing around you, it is affecting people around you, just as their energy is affecting you. A person who is continuously in a negative environment will very quickly become a product of that environment."

Boundaries are extremely important for an empath to feel well, as is connection with nature, movement like yoga, meditation, breath-work, time alone, and grounding. These things are not nice to have; they are essential, non-negotiable rituals for your mental health and wellbeing.

Here is a prayer I use daily to help me manage my energy. I have it in a beautiful print, framed on my bathroom wall, and I say it in the shower every day. You might like it too:

"I ask that anything which is not in my Greatest Good go back to the person it came from, only if it is in their Greatest Good.

If not, I ask that it goes back to Universal Energy or Mother Earth for her cleansing.

I claim my own energetic space."

Read it and see how it makes you feel. If you feel a connection to these words then using this everyday will be helpful to you.

You must take time to understand your identity and create loving boundaries around yourself.

Take steps towards yourself every day.

It is time for you to come home and know yourself at all levels.

Affirmations

- I take time to know who I am on a daily basis
- I live a life aligned to my values
- I accept, honour and love all that I am
- It is safe for me to set boundaries

- I lovingly create space in my life for my own needs and desires

Exercises

What if you simply created a new identity for yourself every day?

Approach each morning with the excitement and newness of a blank sheet of paper and ask: Who do I get to be today? What adventures lie ahead of me today? How can I be of service to the greater good today? How can I honour my needs today?

Practice setting boundaries. Spend time thinking about the following questions and explore where you can start to make shifts towards changing behaviour that is not serving your joy:

- Where are you bleeding energy in places that don't feel good?

- When do you say yes, but really want to say no?

- Do you have expectations in your relationships that you have not communicated? How can you communicate your needs from a place of love?

- Where can you ask for help?

Elicit Your Values

1. Step one: Read through the words below and see which ones you connect with the most.

2. Step two: Identify 10 values, either from the list or other words you consider incredibly important that are not on this list

3. Step three: Identify your top five values out of these 10 – which ones are absolutely the most important to you in life?

4. Step four: Answer the following questions about each of your top five values:

    *   Where do I have alignment to this value in my life?

    *   When do I not have alignment to this value in my life?

    *   What do I need to do to create a life more aligned to this value?

Abundance

Achievement

Acceptance

Authenticity

Balance

Wellbeing

Contentment

Care for Others

Humour

Honesty

Order

Dependability

Quality

Courage

Kindness

Effectiveness

Creativity

Knowledge

Diversity

Empathy

Loyalty

Fun

Excellence

Openness

Innovation

Fairness

Passion

Fitness

Faith

Perseverance

Gratitude

Family

Respect for Others

Simplicity

Freedom

Responsibility

Peace

Friendship

Security

Self-Respect

Generosity

Serenity

Success

Growth

Service to Others

Wisdom

Independence

Spirituality

Discipline

Cooperation

Love

Equality

Stability

Winning

Teamwork

Self-control

Joy

Love is Always the Answer

We all have a limited number of days left on this earth. Each and every one of those days is deeply precious. Your *life* is deeply precious.

If you live until the age of 90, that's 32,850 days in total. So if you're 35, that means that you've got 20,075 days left until you're 90. If you're 45, then there's 16,425 days left until you're 90. If you're 55, there are 12,775 days left until you're 90. And if you're 65, there are 9,125 days left until you're 90.

I'd love you to start thinking about the quality and beauty of your life; reflecting on just how unique and special you really are.

You are capable of *so* much, and the world needs your special talents. It needs you to make the most of your gifts in full. You came here to do that – you came here to grow, learn and expand. We need you in the full and healthy expression of yourself. The more you give yourself permission to shine in the world, the more everyone around you will benefit.

Your life matters so very much. It's incredibly important that you live it from an empowered state where you are making a difference in the world, where you are making a difference in your family, and in your career.

Whenever you feel adrift, listen to your body. Slow down and be grateful for the food that you have and the body you live in. Be mindful. Taste your food. Notice nature around you. Stop and take a breath. Even on the hardest day, there is always something magical to appreciate. Take a moment to slow down and notice what that is.

Make the effort to remove stress from your body. Set goals based on moving forward towards how you want to feel, rather than trying to lose weight. Throw away those scales – they are not doing you any service at all.

You're coming back to your true self by moving towards the vision of health that you've been cultivating. You were never lost. The truth was always there within you. Losing weight is simply an expression of deep love and acceptance of yourself; it will happen with ease as you learn to love who you are and make nourishing choices because you deserve them.

Remember: nurture over punishment. The magic lies in nourishing your body and loving it deeply. Make friends with food and learn how to eat the right foods. Quit trying to burn off unhealthy calories with exercise. Your body just doesn't work like that. Start putting lots of nutrients into your body instead. Eat lots of beans, and legumes, and pulses, and plenty of fibre.

Despite how strange and difficult it may feel, always put yourself first. It is selfless for you to prioritise yourself and put effort into nurturing yourself in thought, in body, and in mind.

As we head into a future in which women are rising into positions of power, it's more important than ever that our self-talk and self-care matches the truth of our biology and empowers us. There is nobody else more invested in our own wellbeing. We owe it to ourselves to step into our own power and educate ourselves in order to flourish and bloom.

Female empowerment starts with being strong and empowered on the inside. It's about achieving unconditional love and acceptance for yourself. It's a monumental shift from thinking you need to reach some external goal in order to be worthy of love, to knowing that you are wholly loveable exactly as you are. But when a woman makes decisions based on the fact that she loves herself rather than a need to be loved by others, she is truly unstoppable.

A woman in her fully empowered state is a beautiful and powerful sight to behold – and everybody around her benefits. When women transform their health and unleash their potential, it pays off in their relationships, parenting, career, and community.

How do we get there? There are many ways. We've looked at mindset. We've looked at setting goals. We've looked at beliefs and values, living in alignment, tuning into your authentic self, and moving out of the ego-based, fear-based brain. We've looked at moving towards love, choosing your thoughts, setting boundaries, and making empowering choices.

You are a magnificent woman – and you have permission to fully express your feminine wisdom, power, and intuition. Live life from your intuition, trust yourself, take courageous steps to honour all that you are and move into the expanded version of yourself that your heart and soul knows is within you.

Make love your focus. Nurture the beautiful body that you live in and give it what it needs. Focus on health, love, joy and nourishment instead of weight, and pay attention to how you talk to yourself. Work on finding your purpose. Give yourself permission to do nothing. Spend time sitting with yourself and tapping into the wisdom within. And if you would like some extra support and guidance along this path, I would be honoured to accompany you in rising to your full potential.

Here's to you, lady. I'm looking forward to seeing you transform your life in the most beautiful way, from the inside out.

It is time for you to undo the shackles.

It is time for you to spread your wings.

It is time for you to soar.

Show the world your true magnificence.

It is your time.

And remember:

Actually, you ARE beautiful.

No, you don't need to lose weight in order to be happy.

You deserve everything wonderful.

Tomorrow is a new day.

You are loved.

You live in a world full of wonder - you simply need to slow down and notice it.

I think you are awesome.

With so much love and light,

Anna xx

Manufactured by Amazon.ca
Bolton, ON

27000749R00129